19.95
net

ADVOCATING TODAY: A Human Service Practitioner's Handbook

ROBERT SUNLEY

FAMILY SERVICE AMERICA

New York

The publication of this book was made possible
in part by a contribution from the North Shore
Unitarian Universalist Veatch Program.

Copyright © 1983 by

Family Service America

44 East 23rd Street, New York, New York 10010

Library of Congress Cataloging in Publication Data

Sunley, Robert
    Advocating today.

    Bibliography: p.
    1.Social service--United States--Handbooks, manuals,
etc.   2. Public Welfare--United States--Handbooks,
manuals, etc.   3. Welfare recipients--United States--
Handbooks, manuals, etc.   4. Public relations--United
States--Social service--Handbooks, manuals, etc.
I. Title.
HV95.S945 1983   362.8'2'068   83-48068
ISBN 0-87304-201-8

Printed in the United States of America

 3

CONTENTS

                                                    Page
Introduction................................   6

1. Advocacy and Advocacy Programs.............   9
   Key Elements...............................   9
   Structure and Operation.................... 10
     Mission, Goals, Objectives, Action Steps 10
     Agency Characteristics................... 14
     Agency Responsibility and Image......... 15
     Participants in Advocacy................ 16

2. Human Resources for Advocacy............... 17
   Sources of Advocacy Participants........... 18
   Problems with Participation................ 22
   Job Functions.............................. 24
   Job Functions - Case Advocacy............. 25
   Job Functions - Case-to-Cause and
     Public Issue Advocacy................... 27
   Training and Elements of a Training Program 28

3. Advocacy Issues: Values and the Selection
     Process.................................. 32
   Values on the National Level.............. 32
   Values at the Local Level................. 35
   The Selection Process..................... 36

4. Advocacy Issues: Examples of Local
     Problems................................. 39
   Characteristics............................ 39

4

                                                          Page

    Examples...................................   41
    Client Rights..............................   42
        Handling...............................   45
        Physical Characteristics...............   45
        Responsiveness.........................   46
        Attitudes..............................   47
        Abuses.................................   48
        Relevance to Specific Client Groups.....   50
        Planning Services for and with Clients..   51
        Administrative Problems.................   54
        Publicizing of Services; Outreach.......   56
        Enforcement............................   58
    Lack of Services...........................   60
    Checklist of Services......................   60

5. Method: The Study..........................   69
    The Study..................................   71
        The Problem............................   71
        Target Organization or System..........   74
        Advocate Organization and Supporting
            Groups.............................   84
        Proposed Change........................   85

6. Method: Planning...........................   87
    Goals......................................   87
    Strategy...................................   89

7. Method: Intervention.......................   97
    Mass Media.................................   98
        The Press..............................   99
        Television............................   100
        Radio.................................   101
    Audiovisual and Other Materials............   102
    Meetings...................................   107
    Formed Groups..............................   109
    Study/Action...............................   113
    Direct Contact with Decision Makers........   117
    Public Opposition..........................   119

Page

8. Advocacy, Politics, and Government......... 127
    The State Legislature..................... 128
        Initiation of the Bill................. 130
        Introduction of the Bill............... 133
        Referral of Bill to Committee.......... 135
        Floor Debate and Action................ 139
        Preceding Steps Repeated in Other House. 140
        Governor's Action...................... 140
        Implementation......................... 141
    The Process Varies........................ 141
    Monitoring Legislative Activity........... 143
    After a Bill Becomes Law.................. 144
    The Environment for Advocacy.............. 146
    Constancy in Change....................... 148
        People in Government................... 148
        Numbers of People...................... 150
        Volunteers Are Important............... 151

9. Method: Other Aspects of Action.......... 152
    Review.................................... 152
    Revision.................................. 153
    Troubleshooting........................... 153

10.Evaluation................................. 157

Notes.. 160

Bibliography................................. 164

INTRODUCTION

The seed for this book was planted in the 1960s - in the turmoil and struggle over poverty, discrimination and segregation, and civil rights. That decade challenged human service agencies to look beyond their clients' individual problems to the forces of society that afflicted them; it demanded their participation in efforts to counteract those forces.

In the spring of 1969, Family Service Association of Nassau County, New York, a member agency of the Family Service Association of America (FSAA), began a family advocacy program and established the position of family advocate. Robert Sunley participated in that step and, a year later, published a definitive article in Social Casework. The article was titled "Family Advocacy: From Case to Cause."[1]

The involvement of family service agencies in advocacy has grown steadily since that time and Sunley has been in the vanguard of the movement. Today advocacy, counseling, and family life education are the principal programs of FSAA. The organization defines family advocacy in these words:

Family Advocacy as practiced in a Family Service Agency is a service directed to improving conditions for families by harnessing expert knowledge of family needs with the commitment to action and the skills to produce necessary change. It involves a process of working in alliance with or on behalf of a family or individual, a group of families, a neighborhood, or a community, to develop strategies for changing institutionalized conditions, systems, or administrative practices that are seen to have a negative effort on individuals and family life. Family Advocacy goals include not only improvement of existing public and voluntary services and their delivery, but also provision of new or changed forms of social utilities...[2]

Robert Sunley is a pioneer in the movement that produced this statement and that today continues to define and perfect the role of advocacy for human service organizations. His book reflects his experience as both a teacher and a practitioner of advocacy.

It also delineates a vision for the future. Sunley goes well beyond his "case to cause" formulation and writes about public issue advocacy with a perception that transcends the specific casework situation. And while his ideas are the creatures of his own experience and other advocacy activities reported in FSAA literature, he has written a book for all human service agencies.

There are many rewards for the reader and user of this book. It is rich in details, in specifics, in examples. It is a book of the hour, for these are times when advocates must be sure of their ground. The family is a political subject as it has never been before. Politics means opposition. Sunley says much about opposition, conflict, and mixed opinion.

I like his precision. He knows the difference between "adversary" and "advocate." He recognizes that many human service organizations are not adversarial by nature, so his suggestions include approaches that do not increase community conflict.

His concepts have depth and sensitivity. For example, he appreciates the power of participation. To Sunley, advocacy is a broadly participatory enterprise. He recognizes that advocacy is complex and his book reflects his awareness that decisions must be made under pressures of time, politics, organizational limitations, and competition for scarce resources. The next decade will move advocacy activities away from the passionate but naive commitment of the 60s into a new level of sophisticated organizational activity. In many ways, Sunley's book introduces that change by integrating individual professional practice, activity by groups of lay people, and established social service agencies. If they want to advocate in ways that work, it is the book they need.

Robert M. Rice

ADVOCACY AND ADVOCACY PROGRAMS

Advocacy is both a social work method and an agency function. As such, it can be embodied in a service, in the total agency structure, or in both.

KEY ELEMENTS

Many definitions of advocacy have been formulated. Although any one definition suffers from the problems inherent in making definitions, there is a consensus on the key elements. These elements also differentiate advocacy from the somewhat related activities of the ombudsman, lawyer, and legislator, and from other social work methods.

These elements are:
A method or process that can be viewed as a part of social work - a planned and purposive change effort composed of study, planning, action, and evaluation - analogous to components in other areas of social work;

A core function of human service agencies, opposition to negative impacts of social institutions and systems on people, individually and in groups (including neighborhoods, communities, ethnic and other groups);

Promotion of measures to support and enhance human life individually and generally;

Engagement of increasing numbers of people,
singly and by groups and organizations, in organized efforts;

A potentially adversarial stance on issues,
on the agency level, movement from "case to
cause" based on the agency's experience with the
problems of the people it serves;

On a broader scale, involvement through various
levels and mechanisms on local, state, and national advocacy issues.

STRUCTURE AND OPERATION

Each agency can adapt advocacy to its own characteristics, reflecting the philosophy of the agency and its conception of its particular services.
Its program, once established, should be periodic-
ally reviewed to determine whether in fact the
place of advocacy in the agency conforms to the
initial intent. This can be judged on the basis of
the proportion of staff time given to advocacy, on
the appearance of advocacy issues on the agenda of
board meetings, and on the extent of community participation in advocacy efforts.

This chapter focuses on general considerations
of the place of advocacy in the agency, and on conceptual adaptations necessary to incorporate fully
the advocacy program as a vital method and service.

Mission, Goals, Objectives, Action Steps

The way in which an agency incorporates advocacy
into its structure is the result of a series of
judgments that ultimately derive from the purpose
of the agency.

The purpose of the agency, or "mission," is its
broadest statement of its relation to society.
From the statement of mission are derived subsidiary statements, variously labeled, but referred to

here as "goals," which again have subsidiary statements termed "objectives." Implementation or action steps are directed toward the accomplishment
of objectives.

Most agencies have a statement of mission in
some form. As the broadest expression of the agency's purpose, the statement is likely to persist
unchanged over many years, although certain program
changes may occur. A statement of mission might
read: "...to provide services to help families
under stress from social or interpersonal problems." Such a statement excludes such other kinds
of services to people as direct provision of medical services, but its scope is wide enough to re-
main unchanged despite seemingly major shifts in an
agency's emphasis. Thus, when one large agency
discontinued direct counseling in favor of advocacy
and other methods, its statement of mission (assuming it read as above) would not need revision.

Goals, though broad, do give specificity to the
mission of the agency by representing targets the
agency strives toward but does not necessarily expect to reach soon. Goals inhere in program and
management, or in other terms, output and input.
Input refers to obtaining resources for agency survival and functioning and to internal management of
the resources; output refers to the agency's services. Although goals may not change rapidly,
shifts in their emphasis or priorities may.

Objectives represent specifics within each goal;
to the extent the objectives are achieved, the
agency sees itself drawing nearer to its goals,
carrying out more fully its mission.

Stephen M. Drezner and William B. McCurdy provide a more specific definition of "objective."
The primary characteristic that defines an objective is that it can be stated in operational

terms. By this we mean that the objective can
be stated in such a way that the extent to which
it is accomplished by programs can be measured
or assessed.[1]

Goals and objectives together constitute a
long-range plan for an agency; a short-range plan
comprises the implementation steps toward each objective, translating it into action, and usually is
formulated in short spans of one to two years.

An example of an implementation step would be
the employment of an Hispanic outreach worker.
This step may be one of several necessary to an objective: developing services to the Hispanic population in the community. This objective may in
turn be one of several necessary to the goal of
providing effective services to underserved groups
in the community.

If a family service agency's statement of mission reads "...to provide counseling service...,"
it would be difficult to place family advocacy and
family education within its goals and objectives,
except as subsidiary functions of counseling rather
than parallel functions. Thus the setting of goals
and objectives in a long-range plan denotes the
agency's sense of priorities. The agency's commitment is shown in its allocation of resources for
actions directed to objectives and goals.

The long-range plan and the structure of the
agency are interconnected. The introduction of advocacy as a new goal, with objectives and implementation steps, requires appropriate reorganization
of the structure, including board, administration,
and staff. The placement of the new function within the structure may influence the extent to which
it is supported by agency resources, and as well
the way it may relate agency structure also bears

upon the selection of advocacy issues, as discussed in chapter 4.

Overall, advocacy may be a separate service or function, either parallel or ancillary to other services, or carried out within existing services and by their staffs, or a combination.

Two structural aspects of advocacy – as a service to other agency services or as a method incorporated into other services – may cause confusion and end in reducing advocacy to a separate, unrelated department or office of the agency. As a service, advocacy may or may not carry out case advocacy functions, but it does provide service to the community in dealing with causes developed from agency cases and in acting on public issues coming to the attention of the agency. As a method, advocacy can be participated in by all staff, granted that case advocacy as conducted by staff is related to the causes and issues of concern to the agency.

The structure of the agency, then, has to provide for linkages among the services, for orientation and training of staff in the advocacy method, for review of practice in this aspect of the agency's work, and for transmission of these activities to the goal-setting body of the agency.

In family service agencies, for example, efforts have been made to develop an integrated service comprising family advocacy, counseling, and family life education.[2] The same staff is involved in all three services, and clients enter for service in any one of the three and move from one to another without formality. Advocacy is focused on "case to cause" on matters of immediate importance to clients, who are often the primary participants in the advocacy activity. This model seems to suit a fairly localized "center" approach, serving in effect a neighborhood or small local community.

Conceivably, an agency could be made up of a number
of such centers, with the central organization
heavily focused on advocacy, supporting local
efforts and extending these efforts onto the larger
scenes.

Although in a number of larger agencies advocacy
as a service is set up with its own staff, in
smaller agencies the service function may be carried by a combination of some agency staff members,
the director, board members, and volunteers, ful-
filling the commitment to advocacy both in the service aspect and in the incorporation of advocacy as
a method (see chapter 3).

Setting of goals and concern with structure may
seem removed from daily practice, but pertinent
questions frequently arise in meetings. Is that
our business? How far do we go on this issue?
Should we respond to this request? Are we putting
too much effort into one type of work? Further,
discrepancies between goals and actual performance
create a dynamic to propel an agency into examining
what it is doing and how. The term "internal advocacy" in effect refers to this dynamic; some of
those within the agency seek to modify those features that impede achievement of goals, or to modify goals in response to community needs, new data,
or rethinking of values.[3]

Agency Characteristics
A number of inherent characteristics of a human
service agency give its advocacy certain qualities:

Continuity. The agency, and therefore its advocacy, are ongoing entities, not ad hoc for a
certain issue and/or a certain period of time,
necessitating the elements of permanence - continuity of effort, development of program, evaluation of activities, for example.

Broad functions. Like the agency itself, the advocate is available for a wide variety of issues and concerns, on the general principle of being related to the agency's special concerns. This allows for a broadly responsive service to the community, for linking up issues and organizations widely, and for taking up matters for which no other organization exists.

Linkage to local community. Through its board of directors and advisory committees, the agency has ongoing links to the community. Many independent advocacy groups have few or no such connections, and lack both the input from the local community and the capacity to mobilize support on issues. They may be unable to respond to new, immediate concerns within the community.

Sanction. The agency has both legal and social sanction for its activities, and uses accepted methods of promoting both social and individual change. This gives a force to its advocacy activities, and assurance to others of the validity of its efforts.

Agency Responsibility and Image

Advocacy appears to be generally consonant with the image of a human service agency as a representative for social concerns in its own community, taking action on problems with which it has firsthand contact through its many clients. In so doing, the agency at the same time undertakes a responsibility for the soundness of its position on an issue and the need for change.

Most agencies have found that their family advocacy programs have gained them wider recognition and acceptance, and that their credibility with minority groups in the community is increased. In a few instances, though, agencies have run into unfavorable receptions. It can be expected that an adversarial role may touch off resistances but careful preparation for the introduction of an advocacy program will avert initial reactions. The selection of issues, position, strategies, and conflictual level are influential factors to be taken into account in communities where opposition is anticipated. (See chapters 6, 7 and 8.)

Participants in Advocacy

As the next chapter indicates, an advocacy effort may entail a variety of individuals and groups whose roles may not always be easy to relate to established organizational patterns. An established structure can readily provide for a new variety of counseling service, for example; the service easily fits the familiar categories of staff and clients, of agency administration and board. In comparison, however, an advocacy campaign may involve all of these groups, the staffs and boards of other agencies, and individuals from the community other than the clients. In addition to a variety of groups and individuals, a variety of relationships exist among them. To work effectively with this complexity, an agency may find that an adjustment of its structure is necessary.

2

HUMAN RESOURCES FOR ADVOCACY

Advocacy encompasses a range of human resources, much broader than those involved in other services of agencies - for instance, counseling and education. For example, in counseling, one or sometimes two staff members work directly with a person or group; no one else, from staff, board, volunteers, or community actually sits in and takes part in the counseling. But in advocacy, other people participate in planning, training, coordination, and action. It is usually desirable, often even necessary, to involve many people in advocacy.

This difference makes it necessary to discuss the potential resources for conducting advocacy, the functions that need to be filled in an advocacy effort, and the ways of matching resources and functions. The discussion identifies two types of human resources: "participants," who are all those involved in an advocacy action except for paid workers of the agency, and those workers who are referred to as "staff" or "staff members."

An agency need not assign one staff member solely to advocacy, since the job functions can be divided among various persons and groups. A staff member assigned part-time to be in charge of an advocacy action may be likened to an orchestra conductor who directs many players rather than to a sole performer. Unlike the orchestra players,

however, advocacy participants can carry out much
of the work without the presence of a staff member.

Some agencies hesitate to move from case advocacy into case-to-cause and issue advocacy because
they lack an advocacy staff position. A planned
use of available associates can maximize use of
staff time. In some agencies this is done on a
part-time and ad hoc basis by the executive director or a staff member in relation to each advocacy
effort. A full-time advocate position simply ex-
pands greatly the scope of the agency's advocacy
thrust.

SOURCES OF ADVOCACY PARTICIPANTS
The main sources of advocacy participants are:
Board of Directors
Volunteers
Consumers (including agency clients)
Outside groups (agencies, formal, and informal
  groups)
The staff sources are:
Executive director
Professionals
Paraprofessionals
Clerical and other staff members
Students

The following are specific considerations regarding each source:
Board of Directors. While all board members by
virtue of their joining the board have an interest in social problems, not all wish to be
directly involved in advocacy. Those with a
direct interest form the pool from which an advocacy committee (public issues committee, social concerns committee) may be established and
maintained. Those not on such a committee, however, should not be disregarded. Some may be
able to assist at times by providing contacts or
information. Some may wish to be involved in

one action but not in others. It is desirable,
therefore, to apprise the board of each planned
action in order to enlist help (as well as to
provide accountability for advocacy). As board
members feel needed in advocacy efforts, they
are more likely to be drawn into ongoing support
and into the committee.

Board members of a committee are typically involved in policy matters regarding advocacy, in
assessment on community needs, in broad planning
for action. Individual committee members may
take part in a given effort, and sometimes the
committee as a whole may take up an advocacy
project. As committee members become more aware
of the tasks needed in advocacy, they may volunteer for particular jobs within the overall effort.

Volunteers. These are community people who have
an interest either in a specific advocacy effort
or in an ongoing capacity for advocacy. Volunteers obviously can fill a variety of jobs, depending on training, interest, and ability.
Also, trained volunteers can be especially valuable in case advocacy services, handling many of
the concrete advocacy problems under staff
supervision. Recruitment of volunteers for advocacy can be done in various ways. Agencies
with an ongoing volunteer program often find
that new volunteers come by word of mouth from
currently active volunteers. Other methods include talks before community groups (churches,
civic organizations, for example), fliers, advertisements, and other media presentations. As
with any type of volunteer activity, however,
the orientation, training, and job placement of
volunteers are crucial both in retaining volunteers and in eliciting commitment and effort.
Volunteers may at some point serve as members of
the advocacy committee or may be drawn into

advocacy work from other tasks. Volunteers are also important because they can bring points of view different from those of staff, clients, or board. Some may know particular communities or groups well; others may understand how to appeal to people neutral or antagonistic to the advocacy effort; others may advise on how to present matters in everyday language, or how to recruit more volunteers. Needed expertise may be obtained by recruiting people with specialized knowledge and experience, such as lawyers, doctors, urban planners, housing experts.

Consumers. This refers to those who have the problem. Often they are agency clients who present individual complaints for case advocacy action; the agency puts their complaints together into a case-to-cause action. Frequently such consumers are brought together in a group to take part in an action; they become, in effect, advocacy personnel available to take on certain tasks. The agency seeks consumers in regard to a particular problem, or an already formed group may request the agency's help in carrying out advocacy in its behalf. As with volunteers, the agency has a responsibility for orientation and training in relation to the advocacy process; this may be particularly important in relation to consumers' expectations of the agency and of the process. The agency should give special attention to interconnecting consumers with others involved in an advocacy action, and to the roles that consumers wish to play, avoiding the dangers of both taking over from the consumers and of providing too little support, consultation, or joint effort.

The agency should take note, in proposing advocacy functions for consumers, of the kinds of activity that might afford personal enhancement for the individual consumer. The overt issue-

orientation of advocacy should not obscure the
fact that an advocacy action is made up of individuals (whether board, staff, volunteers, or
consumers) who are going through an important
personal experience. The agency must help make
the experience meaningful for the individual;
this may at times point to the need for consultation with counseling staff.

Outside groups. These include social agencies,
community organizations, formal or informal community groups, and church groups. Usually people from outside the agency become involved if
their organization is involved, either in an ongoing relationship or on an ad hoc basis.
Usually some division of labor occurs in such
collaborative efforts, with the agency providing
only one part. These considerations are important in the planning and organizing phases of an
advocacy effort, and have a bearing on the decision about involving other organizations and
groups.

The following pertains to the use of staff:
Executive director. While the extent of the
executive's involvement varies from agency to
agency and from one advocacy project to another,
the role of the executive is always a key one.
The reason is that the advocacy function is inherently a central function of the agency rather
than solely or primarily a departmental function. It involves board directly or indirectly;
it requires the allocation of agency personnel
from various parts of the agency; it represents
the agency publicly; and it encompasses interests broader than those of any one department or
service of the agency.

In agencies with a family advocate, the executive usually is less directly involved in advocacy action but maintains the overall responsi-

bility through conferences with the advocate and
through liaison with the board and the advocacy
committee. Where the advocate functions are
taken up by one or more staff members, the executive again participates indirectly. Whatever
the arrangement, the executive director must
keep in touch with the movement of an advocacy
effort.

Agency staff. Staff available for advocacy includes professionals, paraprofessionals, clerical and other staff, and students. The job
functions required in an advocacy effort, described below, indicate an inclusive and differential use of staff members. Staff not usually
thought of as contributing to an advocacy effort
may be drawn in. A person specializing in family life education may be used in training of
volunteers because of his or her expertise in
working with groups. Clerical staff members may
receive specific assignments, depending on interest, capability, and availability; they
should be regarded as part of the advocacy staff
and brought into orientation and training sessions so that they can deepen their understanding and their contribution. For agencies with a
small staff, graduate social work students
studying community organization can carry out
several advocacy functions.

PROBLEMS WITH PARTICIPATION

One of the most frequently encountered problems
is that of developing and maintaining the involvement of a sufficient number of consumers in a given
advocacy effort. The same may be said of all kinds
of participants. Two or three consumers, for example, may be very involved and determined, but they
and the advocate find it difficult to bring in more
participants. The best single source of help on
this problem is the chapter, "Fostering Participation," in Rothman's book Promoting Innovation and

Change in Organizations and Communities.[1] He develops several principles based on research, with a
particular focus on the involvement of low-income
persons. He describes two main types of benefits
that foster participation: instrumental, providing
material or tangible returns; and expressive, providing psychological benefits such as friendships,
personal satisfaction, and pride. He then gives
examples of how the principles were tried out in
action, with comments from the advocates.

The fostering of participation is thus of high
importance at the beginning of an advocacy effort,
but needs to be maintained and further developed
during the entire effort. As much consideration
must be given to participation as to the development of the advocacy issue and the use of intervention techniques.

Other factors impeding participation include:
The selection of the advocacy issue. Broad issues that are difficult to tackle and require a
long-term effort may discourage participation,
since tangible results are often long delayed,
if they occur at all. Local issues may be more
achievable and hence may foster better and
broader participation. For example, the study
and clarification of a welfare issue may show
that both local and state-wide issues are involved. A group of welfare recipients may have
a range of complaints, from the way they are
treated at the local office to the amount of al-
lotment. The former issue can be approached
more directly by the group, which encourages
participation. Members of the group can usually
have a more active and direct part in the advocacy effort, and enjoy a solid sense of accomplishment. Participation in the broader issue
may then be fostered for at least some members
of the group.

Adverse conditions surrounding the advocacy effort. These may involve such down-to-earth factors as distance to the meeting place and transportation problems; inconvenient meeting times;
lack of child-care; feeling uncomfortable in the
agency setting; concern about hidden agenda of
the agency or staff; disappointment remaining
from earlier involvement in social action; concern about racial or other bias in the agency.

Pace. Some participants may feel left behind,
not "on board," as if they had come in the middle of the activity. This may lead to the feeling of not belonging, of not being able to contribute, of not obtaining any satisfaction from
being present.

Change in circumstances. When some participants
happen to drop out for unavoidable reasons, the
remaining participants may interpret this as
lack of conviction, which in turn weakens their
own sense of purpose.

JOB FUNCTIONS

The principal job functions in advocacy actions
are listed below. As noted previously, the types
of staff and advocacy participants sought should be
related to the tasks required to carry out the action.

Planning. Clarification of problem; gathering
data; analysis of data; development of initial
plan.

Organizing. Outlining action steps in terms of
staff and associates; recruitment of associates,
with interpretation of the problem, the data,
the agency, the roles, the goals.

Training. Preparing for action; developing
skills, knowledge, attitudes, commitment.

Direction and coordination. Coordination and supervision of those involved; for example, evaluating action steps for possible revision.

Arranging. Setting up details of meetings; preparation and production of materials; other support services.

Advocating. Includes all the action steps - phone calls, letters, petitions, participating in meetings, acting as spokesman, for example.

JOB FUNCTIONS - CASE ADVOCACY

This section deals with the case advocacy part of case-to-cause, in which the primary relationship is between an advocate and an individual or family.

Planning. Worker and client share this role, though the client's participation in this and subsequent stages will vary, depending on such factors as present capability, other pressures, physical limitations, etc. For example, with a very frail or disoriented elderly person, the worker may have to take on virtually the entire process alone. In any event, the worker should go through each part of the planning phase, and this may require including others in the planning - agency staff or staff from other organizations, for example.

Organizing. This may apply in case advocacy when the worker needs to involve the whole family (or extended family) by interpreting the problem, the target, the plan of action, and possible risks, in order to enlist support and possible participation.

Training. This function may be minimal, but often the worker may need to prepare the client through role playing, discussion, etc., for playing the advocate role in meeting the target institution. The client may also need help with the required knowledge, in clarifying the problem and exploring risks. The elements of training for a case advocate are outlined below. In some agencies, a separate service and/or specific staff member is designated to handle case advocacy problems for people who approach the agency for help with only those problems (that is, they are not people applying for counseling). In such a service, training of case advocates, whether staff or volunteers, is an important part of the advocacy process.

Direction/coordination. The relative roles of client and worker again will vary. Often the worker, because of more knowledge and experience in similar situations, may be the coordinator. However, to the extent possible, the worker will encourage the client to take on this function, with the worker acting more as a consultant.

Arranging. This function may require the involvement of other agency personnel: letters to be written, documents photocopied, forms completed, etc.

Advocating. While it may be the ideal for the client to act as advocate, many situations are crises and it may well be more important to obtain a favorable resolution by having the worker present in some capacity than to hope that the client will profit by acting independently. The worker should be alert, however, to such situations, since they are prime "cause" advocacy situations; when the worker's presence is needed for the client to be treated fairly or decently, it can be assumed that other people have had adverse experiences also. Whether or not the crisis situation permits of delay until a cause group can be developed, the worker should help the client understand that the agency will try to make this experience, along with others, into an action helpful to others.

JOB FUNCTIONS - CASE-TO-CAUSE AND
PUBLIC ISSUE ADVOCACY

This section relates job functions to both case-to-cause and public issues advocacy.

Planning. Generally, some initial planning takes place, usually within a relatively small group. A worker with a small group of clients with a common problem may develop an initial plan which leads into organizing - bringing others into the advocacy effort. This leads again into further planning with the larger group. Or, as another example, staff may have gathered data from the caseload, developed an initial plan, and then brought in clients and others. Beyond this initial planning, however, advocacy often requires further organizing, recruiting, and training of others, and developing ties with other organized groups with similar interests. The planning stage is crucial, since the knowledge base must be prepared and analyzed in order to recruit advocacy associates. The plan must be elaborated sufficiently so that the relevant associates can be involved to prepare for action.

Organizing. As indicated, this stage is interwoven with the planning stage. In organizing, the initial approaches are made to other groups and organizations and they are brought in on further planning. Often a staff member carries the primary responsibility for the planning and organizing stages, but this does not preclude delegation of much of the work to others. Participants, including clents, may work on obtaining the needed data, with the staff member giving guidance in what needs to be obtained and where. Also, the staff member may be the one to

make initial contacts with other groups, but in
actual meetings, associates may carry out the
process of orienting newcomers and bringing them
into the planning and organizing.

Training and elements of a training program.
The extent of training may range from ad hoc
training for a small group for a one-time advocacy effort to a formalized training program to
develop an ongoing pool of advocates. Generally, if an agency is going to continue in advocacy, some form of training program becomes desirable to provide the various types of advocacy
participants and staff with basic knowledge,
skills, and attitudes. However, many cause efforts involving small client groups will of necessity require ad hoc training for each group.
In these situations, experienced volunteers or
student advocates can provide much of the training.

A training program should consist of several
general elements, which can be varied or modified according to the people to be trained and
the situations or purposes:

1) Advocacy. Its nature, nature of agency, advocacy roles, process of advocacy.

2) Concerns.   Possible targets of advocacy,
   goals of advocacy in relation to problems;
   client and consumer groups to benefit from
   action.

3) Experiential. Field visits, contacts with
   client and other groups; field work (such as
   court monitoring); observation of advocacy
   activity in agency. In some agencies, service programs to provide case advocacy experience may be set up; trainees can gain understanding and commitment by participating in
   such services.

4) Sensitivity. Attention must be paid to the trainee's own feelings and attitudes - toward the poor, minorities, the elderly. This applies also to training of client groups, who may have adverse feelings and attitudes, not only about others, but also about themselves. Usually this part of the training is best done in small groups with a trainer, so that airing of feelings, sharing of attitudes, and some group development can occur. The need for this part of training tends to merge out of the previous steps, as trainees themselves begin to recognize where they are in relation to the process. The trainer helps the group move in this direction, rather than imposing such training arbitrarily or prematurely because "they need it." Lack of attention to this part of training may well result in weak commitment, dissension, and distortion of objectives, for example. Agency staff experienced in work with groups can help directly, or indirectly through consultation with the trainer.

5) Knowledge. The focus and extent will vary according to the type of training. In cause advocacy involving a small group on an ad hoc basis, the knowledge base may be relatively limited - information on the target institution, the laws, regulations, practices, structure, relating to the specific problem. Trainees should also know about other efforts made in the past, and the nature and interests of other organizations connected with the cause.

In a formalized training program, trainees would receive an orientation to the various helping systems and their development - criminal justice, health, mental health, and income support, for example.

Direction/coordination. This is obviously a key function, and one that evolves from the beginning of an advocacy effort. It is not essential, however, that the same person or persons have this role from the beginning. In the planning stage, for example, others may carry the main responsibility and work, and at a somewhat later point the executive or coordinating function may be more formally established, with different people. In small-scale cause actions, a staff member may carry this function from the beginning. In large-scale efforts, however, such as those involving the development of coalitions, the structure may be established later. Common patterns of structure then usually locate the directive and coordinative function in an executive committee or steering committee, with or without designated chairpersons. For example, a simple organizational structure comprised of committees and a general membership establish an executive committee made up of committee chairpersons. Whatever the structure, certain executive and coordinative functions must be carried out; one of the most important is that of making quick decisions or responses, and usually this responsibility is delegated to the executive group or person.

It is important that one or more individuals be in a position to understand and work with the totality of the advocacy action. This function includes evaluation of where the weaknesses of the action are, what new groups may need to be involved, whether new forms of action may be needed. Such persons, though not necessarily making the decisions, must be in a position to call meetings and present the need for change. The function of spokesman, included under the heading of "Advocating" below, is also usually carried out by one or more persons with directive or coordinative responsibility.

Arranging. This function can often be handled largely by volunteers. It involves such time-consuming but vital matters as getting advocacy participants to meetings, arranging times, transportation, and any other supports, preparation of materials, and distributing them to the people who will use them.

Advocating. In this stage, various staff and advocacy associates may be needed. In large-scale efforts, people may be required to get petitions signed, distribute fliers and posters, send out letters, make phone calls. Other activities include meetings of various kinds, from small ones between advocates and representatives of an institution to large public meetings or demonstrations.

The function of spokesman is included here. It involves representing the advocacy action to the media (TV, radio, newspapers) and at meetings and conferences. Often part or all of this function can be carried out by trained and experienced volunteer advocates or client spokesmen.

Participation in the advocating function is particularly important for client groups. Their visibility and firsthand knowledge of the problem are extremely effective in bringing about change, and their participation reduces feelings of helplessness and alienation.

3

ADVOCACY ISSUES: VALUES AND THE SELECTION PROCESS

At any one time there is a multitude of issues on which an agency could take action, whether local, state, or national in scope. Selection of certain issues, then, involves not only consideration of data, but, more importantly, brings into play many values - those of the broad society, of human service agencies, and of the participating individuals (board, staff, consumers of agency services, and community people). Values enter in as the number of issues is narrowed down; values enter as well into the study, planning and implementation of advocacy efforts. Awareness of values and of conflicts among values must then always be a concern of those involved; the establishment and functioning of adequate selection mechanisms are also vital, both to reconcile value conflicts and to foster openness to newly developing or emerging values.

VALUES ON THE NATIONAL LEVEL

For example, society has placed high value upon the family, as the unit that rears children, instilling values and socialization, and as a basic economic and emotional support system for its members. A major expression of this value is the vast array of social programs aimed at families or aspects of family life. Yet such programming at the same time tends to have unforeseen negative impacts

upon family life or upon some groups, running counter to other highly held values in our culture.

As one example, the rights of the individual
have been heavily stressed from the earliest days
of our government. According to Robert M. Rice,
"...The United States Constitution is silent on the
subject of the family...The system of inherited
social status, so much a part of the English monar-
chy of the time, was to be avoided in the new American society. The possibility that the family
might occupy central attention with the American
Constitution posed the problem of the maintenance
of a nobility."[1] Family law thus became a matter
for the different states, and social welfare services followed this pattern, resulting in a patch-
work without a central national focus on the family. Conflicts about family versus individual
value systems erupt frequently, as in the rights of
children against the rights of parents, in the
rights of the mentally ill against the family and
local interests, in the rights of women against
long-held beliefs in the roles of men and women in
the family.

Another closely related value is that of the
sanctity of the family, of its integrity against
intrusions by the government. Such intrusions may
be experienced as social programs that run counter
to group beliefs and values, infringing upon family
relationships, or as programs that weaken the family structure or seem to foster dependency upon
government allotments rather than encouraging
self-help.[2]

The literature on values points up a change in
the conception of values. Once there were values -
the "good" - that were considered eternal, but now
values are seen to differ according to a social and
temporal context. Following the latter trend, family advocacy values can be directly related to our

own social context, and more specifically to such developments as the vast proliferation of government benefits, restrictions, and regulations since World War II. In this light, family advocacy tries to assist families to maintain their position as against malfunctioning aspects of government and to press for improvements or for nongovernmental movements and measures. Government in turn may be seen as the mediator among the many conflicting forces within society, with family advocacy helping the less powerful groups to influence the mediator in their behalf, as well as to counteract negative impacts from the government itself.

Such advocacy rests upon certain other values widely held in our society. One such value stems from the egalitarian aim of our society - to provide equal rights and fair treatment for all. Advocacy upholds this value in seeking to redress wrongs and remedy deficiencies. Another such value is that of participatory democracy, in which each person is entitled to engage in efforts to bring about equality or promote beneficial change. Participation in advocacy, then, is not limited to certain groups or professionals, but is open to anyone interested in a cause. Advocacy in behalf of human welfare thus implies the participation of many in an effort to realize further some of our society's major values. Family advocacy engages forces to promote the welfare of families, not at the expense of individuals, but to enlarge governmental and public concern with the family as a key social unit.

A value contained within advocacy is that action directed toward a social goal is itself constructive, in contrast to passive acceptance of authority. Family advocacy as social action becomes a means of helping individuals, above and beyond such direct individual help as counseling. A judgment is implied that help to the individual is not sufficient to meet all needs, that there are impacts upon individuals and families that cannot and should not be countered only by separate individual adaptations.

VALUES AT THE LOCAL LEVEL

The values that enter into the selection and ordering of possible issues for action are not only the broad values of concern to advocates. Value judgments in the selection of issues are also made by the participating individuals and groups, and resolution of their conflicting values at times becomes an essential part of the advocacy process.

For example, a particular measure for welfare reform may be differently viewed by groups involved in advocacy, though all hold the same basic values. Positions may also change over time, due to additional data, as well as insights on the consequences of a given measure or method. This has been particularly evident in recent years, when the biases widespread in our society against blacks, Hispanics, the poor, the aged, and other groups have been brought into the open largely through advocacy efforts from those groups and allied advocacy organizations. Those making decisions in advocacy would need to be generally in accord with agency philosophy.

A group encountering difficulties in reaching agreement on issues may use various methods to elicit value positions and then move the entire group to a resolution of variances. For example, the Delphi method elicits and refines group values and is designed to counteract the frequent negative features of group process: the biasing effect of dominant individuals, irrelevant communications, and group pressure toward conformity. The method utilizes a formal anonymous questionnaire with findings presented statistically, extending over several sessions to elicit feedback and allow for

individual changes until the final summing up.
This and other methods, from simple to complex, are
described in "A Planning Guide," by Drezner and
McCurdy.[3]

Social work staff members must relate to the
values of their professional organization which can
conceivably come into conflict with other values,
especially as to the professional principle of
holding the client's welfare to be primary, above
that of agency or other interests.[4] This may run
counter to the position of an agency that does not
carry out or subscribe to advocacy; staff may experience a constraint against assisting clients
with advocacy, whether on a case or cause level.
In the family service field, a major step toward
overcoming such conflict occurred with Family Service Association of America recognized advocacy as
a major function of family agencies and required
specific advocacy activity as a requirement for accreditation. This move strengthened the positions
of individual social workers, advocacy committees,
and agencies themselves in relation to funding organizations.

THE SELECTION PROCESS

Agencies with an advocacy program develop a
mechanism for the selection of advocacy issues.
Frequently, an advocacy committee is set up, composed of board members and usually the executive
director and staff members. Sometimes, nonagency
people sit on the committee as individuals or as
representatives of groups.

One task of the committee is to conduct regular
reviews of problems in the community, obtaining information from staff and outside sources. A helpful guide is the comprehensive checklist of services provided in chapter 4.

The committee also needs a means of involving the entire agency in the case-to-cause process, thus bringing to the committee the cause issues relating to the services the agency provides - those issues affecting more than one individual. This information must be gathered at the case service level, with staff processing the multitude of case advocacy efforts into causes. Some agencies have developed sophisticated methods of obtaining such information from service staff, which involves staff thoroughly in the advocacy process.

Through its minutes and reports at board meetings, the committee maintains its responsibility to the board and obtains overall direction.

Although the structure within which an advocacy program operates may vary from agency to agency, the mechanisms must provide for expression of a wide range of opinion and values. Selection of issues must develop out of broad consideration of both issues and the agency's goals and objectives.

Some agencies have developed criteria for selecting advocacy issues, including:
- number of people affected by the problem
- severity of the effects of the problem
- capability of the agency to tackle the problem
- extent to which other groups are involved in working on the problem
- probability of making an impact upon the problem
- length of time probably needed to have impact
- constraints possibly involved in a given issue
- extent of outside support needed
- timeliness of issue in the community

Data can be obtained on several of these factors, but obviously represent only one basis for

the judgments that must be made. Other factors require input from staff and from outside the agency,
as well as decisions as to the effect on the agency's resources. The agency also needs balance in
allocating efforts to local issues as against
broader issues in which it may be joining with many
other organizations on state or national matters.

An analysis of advocacy issues shows that about
half of the issues could be categorized as local
and half as state, regional, and national. This
does not, however, indicate the allocation of issues within any one agency, nor does it indicate
the proportions of effort and time expended.[5]

As an agency gains experience in advocacy efforts, it becomes better able to evaluate some of
the factors needed, such as capability, constraints, and length of time and kind of effort
required.

The selection of issues for advocacy may be
termed "intake" in analogy to the intake policies
and practices of a counseling service. Many of the
same concerns and considerations enter into both;
both are crucial in that they are the points at
which the value judgments, philosophy, and commitment of an agency are brought to bear for decision
making. These decisions also show a community what
an agency stands for.

4

ADVOCACY ISSUES: EXAMPLES OF LOCAL PROBLEMS

Local problems are those in which the power to make change resides in local government or local organizations. This is in contrast to problems which, though affecting people locally, can be remedied only through action on a state or federal level. The latter problems usually require broad effort by many organizations; the single action of firing off letters or board resolutions to a governor or legislator is quite ineffectual.

CHARACTERISTICS

Local problems can surface to agency awareness through case-to-cause or as public issues. They are important targets for advocacy, particularly for small agencies and for agencies developing an advocacy program, as the following points show:

Smaller scale. Local problems usually require a small-scale mobilization of forces, and many local problems can be handled by an agency that has relatively few resources for advocacy.

Participation of clients. Local problems are such that clients can often be involved throughout the advocacy process. A client group may be the primary advocacy force involved, giving clients a stronger sense of acting in their own behalf (in contrast to being involved in a statewide effort, for example, where many groups converge and most clients may participate only marginally or in mass demonstrations).

Access to decision makers. Generally, local decision makers can be readily identified as one or a few specific people; usually the agency can gain access to such decision makers in person. Also, persons and groups with influence on decision makers can be identified and worked with. This contrasts with problems on state and federal levels, where the decision makers are many and at various levels and lines of power and influence are varied and complex.

Shorter time frame. Local problems are generally susceptible of being resolved much sooner than state or federal problems. This is important in regard to recruiting and using various sources of manpower for advocacy. It is important also for clients, board, and staff to achieve results quickly in order to sense the movement of advocacy and the satisfaction of success.

Publicity. Local media are often more accessible to advocacy actions on local problems, and the agency is in a good position to be regarded as having expertise on such problems. Such publicity, beyond its usefulness for the problem at hand, helps the agency to make its services known to the community and to potential clients, and to establish the agency as functioning broadly to help the community.

Level of expertise. This refers to the knowledge base and the data needed in a given action. Client and volunteer groups often can make effective studies of local problems, but would have much more difficulty with a state or federal issue requiring extensive data and expertise in several areas.

The foregoing points do not mean, however, that advocacy on local problems is easy compared to that directed to state and federal problems. Some local problems are relatively simple and straightforward but others may be quite complex and difficult. A local issue may provoke more dissension on an agency board than many broader issues removed from direct local impact.

State and federal problems obviously involve consequences to large populations, often in relation to very basic needs - for example, the level of income maintenance for public assistance. While legislative changes appear more permanent and enforceable than local changes, the many levels of bureaucracy involved in implementing change may well present further problems. Also, legislation may be ambiguous, contradictory, or defective in certain aspects, again giving rise to a new cycle of problems requiring advocacy action. Court action on a state or federal level, though broad in scope and effect, may not have conclusive results on a practice level.

Many local problems exist because the systems intended to deal with them are ineffective. Agencies most frequently give their attention to problems within social service systems. However, dysfunctions obviously occur in other systems, with direct impact on people in need of help - in cultural and recreational activities, in business and industry, in environmental control, for example. It is important for an agency to be aware of such problems and include them in the totality of potential advocacy situations to be considered and placed in its order of priorities.

EXAMPLES

To understand the variety of operational problems that result from ineffective service, it is helpful to categorize them according to special characteristics and to consider examples. This analysis also provides a framework for studying a given organization in order to expand the advocacy action. For example, an agency received complaints from clients about long delays at a certain organization. A study revealed other administrative problems and poor planning of services. The one advocacy action was therefore aimed at improvements beyond those sought in the single presenting complaint.

CLIENT RIGHTS

Rights, as used here, refers to specific, defined rights or entitlements under law or governmental regulations. It does not include broad humanitarian concepts such as a client's right to be treated decently, or even more generally, the right to an adequate income. It is usually advisable to have legal opinion on whether a right is involved in a given situation.

Advocacy questions pertinent in this area are:
. Is the client's right being obviously disregarded? (See example 1, which follows)
. Is there disagreement whether client's situation falls within the right? (example 2)
. Are the facts about the client's situation in dispute? (example 3)
. Are there conflicting laws and regulations? (example 4)

In terms of local issues, the advocate can play some role in all of these kinds of problems, although the last one especially may remove the issue from a local to a judicial or state or federal level. However, the advocate working with clients can endeavor to resolve issues of rights with the local institution (usually governmental) through pertinent advocacy methods. Problems involving rights may at times require legal intervention and court resolution; the advocate's role, beyond initial efforts to resolve the problem without legal recourse, may be in providing support to the client, assistance in gathering information, and development of a client group with the same problem, as in examples 1 and 5.

While there may be a legal basis for advocating for a right in the courts, the process requires extensive documentation that may be difficult to get; also, the outcome of recourse to the courts is uncertain. Hence, the action of the advocate may in many situations be preferable, as illustrated in examples 5 and 6.

Example 1: The client was receiving SSI benefit lower than the current public assistance level. The advocate helped the client apply for assistance, but the application was rejected and conferences with the Department of Social Services were unsuccessful. Many other cases existed. The client was referred to free legal service, which took up the case and fought it through the courts, with final success.

Example 2: In one community, applicants for Emergency Assistance for Adults (EAA) were almost uniformly denied help. An advocate surveyed conditions in comparable communities in the state and indicated that local clients were relatively disadvantaged. The local Department of Social Services (DSS), however, contended that these applicants did not meet the requirements for EAA, not that DSS was failing to utilize the law and regulations permitting grants.

Example 3: An elderly woman came to the agency in despair; her SSI benefits had just been greatly reduced, to the point where she could not both pay rent and eat. Investigation by an advocate revealed that her landlord, an old friend, had given the governmental office an overly high estimate of the value of her lodgings, thinking to do her a favor; also in her application she referred to receiving money from relatives. Under the regulations, receipt of these outside benefits required a corresponding reduction in payments. The advocate obtained statements to show the market value of her lodgings and statements from relatives showing they had not actually contributed regular support. The advocate began to document other cases with the same problem.

Example 4: Several participants in a public assistance work program complained they had been cut off for 90 days for failing to report for work; they claimed they had reported and had been told there was no work on those days. There was no appeal mechanism provided for this situation. While it appeared that a right may have been violated by this procedure, the advocate instead appealed to the government agency, pointing out that the participants in the program did not have any record form on which it could be noted that they had reported (if such were the case). Other governmental programs were cited in which participants retain a card on which entries are made and signed by the supervisor, and in which appeal mechanisms were provided.

Example 5: A local community hospital seemed to be following discriminatory practices in its staffing patterns, with no minority people on staff except in lowest level positions. Rather than attempt to prepare documentation necessary for legal action, the advocate appeared before a hospital accreditation hearing with a client group and testified to the problem. The resulting publicity brought about a change in hospital staffing.

Example 6: Through an agency's outreach program, the advocate learned that a number of persons were failing to receive service from a local treatment facility due to elaborate admis-
sion procedures including completion of a lengthy questionnaire mailed to them at home. Staff
of the facility resisted an appeal for change.
While it appeared that a right to service was
being violated, the law and regulations were not
specific and recourse to the courts would be
necessary to enforce the right. An appeal by
the advocate to the governing board of the facility, pointing out the consequences of the policies to the individuals and to the community,
brought about a change.

Handling

The actual daily points of contact between an
institution and its clients provide many occasions
for advocacy. On one hand, this is an area generally least susceptible to legislation, regulation,
or legal means for correction; it commands perhaps
the least attention, in part because it does not
usually involve large issues attracting publicity.
On the other hand, the institution generally has in
itself the power to correct the problem. Hence it
is a major area for case and case-to-cause advocacy.

For purposes of clarity, the description of the
handling of clients in subsequent paragraphs has
been divided into several categories: physical
characteristics of the institution, responsiveness
to clients, attitudes of staff toward clients, and
abuses of clients. The following examples under
each grouping, while not exhausting the possibilities, give the nature and range of the problems encountered:

Physical characteristics

Example 1: When the local Department of Social
Services moved to a new building, with provision

for interviewing offices, adequate waiting room, etc., clients soon made known a major valid complaint: The new location was far removed from access by public transportation. Clients had to embark on a series of bus trips plus a taxi to get there; both in terms of time expended and cost, clients were suffering. The advocate proposed a plan for satellite offices and outpost workers, after documenting the problem.

Example 2: After a local agency started a program of lay advocates to accompany clients to the Department of Social Services, the agency found there were serious problems regarding the waiting room. It was so small that clients often had to stand for hours, was poorly ventilated, lacked any play area for children, and provided no way by which clients could obtain food on the premises. Not only did clients have to arrive early in the morning and wait for hours, but some were dismissed in the afternoon because the staff could not get to them that day.

Example 3: In a similar situation, an agency found that the department had no public telephones available to clients who might need to call home or call for information.

Example 4: In still another situation, advocates found little or no privacy for interviewing most clients; a few cubicles were provided, but clients often were interviewed in the waiting room because of overcrowding.

Responsiveness
Example 1: On the basis of information from staff, the advocate found that private agencies in the community were not providing evening hour availability for working people, and brought together agency representatives.

Example 2: SSI clients complained to an agency
that they were told, when their checks failed to
arrive, that they didn't need to worry; they
would get their checks. But they could not get
an estimate of how long it would take. The advocate found that SSI staff did not recognize
that the clients were anxious and had to plan
for survival, and that remedying errors was ur-
gent.

Example 3: The agency staff and clients complained that it often took days for the Department of Social Services to answer a phone call.
Clients without phones had given up making calls
from pay phones, since they could not reach anyone and couldn't be called back. Investigation
showed that the problem was partly due to an
acute shortage of phones in the DSS offices and
partly to low staff morale which was reflected
in disregard of clients.

Attitudes
Example 1: Teenagers in one community complained that police consistently harassed them,
breaking up groups that formed in public places,
picking up teenagers, manhandling them, and in-
sulting them in an effort to track down van-
dals. Teenagers in cars complained that police
routinely pulled them over and searched them and
their cars, sometimes in front of neighbors.
The advocate gathered information from youth
workers in the community and then proposed a
plan of education for the police and a plan for
community facilities for youth.

Example 2: Through a program of visits to a
nursing home by volunteers, the agency learned
that elderly patients felt they got perfunctory
medical care and little attention from staff.
Exploration revealed that the staff regarded
patients as hopeless and troublesome and did not
feel the need to give real care.

48

Example 3: From repeated cases, the agency learned that one judge in the family court consistently rejected women's complaints about physical violence from their husbands, placing the blame on women and insisting that they put up with the situations. The advocate worked with the presiding judge and the local Bar Association to bring pressure to bear on this judge.

Example 4: Minority clients complained of treatment at the local Department of Social Services: receptionists were rude, unhelpful; they could see staff members laughing about them; staff members gave them legalistic explanations without any effort to explain fully; if they persisted they were considered troublemakers and made to wait longer or arbitrarily dismissed. Investigation, including contacts with some DSS staff, bore out the substance of the complaints. A client group, with the advocate, met with the administration to press for changes.

Example 5: The agency received many complaints from clients and staff about practices in the emergency room of a large urban hospital. Some were turned away; others waited excessively long hours for emergency help for wounds. All complained that many doctors spoke and understood English so poorly that clients were bewildered and uncertain what to do. Those not on Medicaid reported that unless they could pay cash in advance for the emergency room fees, they were turned away. Clients, advocates, and an interested reporter met with the hospital administration and obtained assurances of changes.

Abuses
Example 1: Agency staff members reported several instances of foster children, removed from their own homes because of abuse, being physically and sexually abused in foster homes.

Contacts with agencies furnished additional
data, and the advocate and board members met
with the foster care staff to press for improved
supervision of foster children.

Example 2: Through contacts with relatives of
elderly people in a local nursing home, staff
learned of serious abuses - attendants punching
patients, threatening them with being put out,
unnecessarily confining patients in rooms, tying
them down, punishing them by withholding care or
food. The agency spearheaded the formation of a
coalition of concerned organizations to press
for changes in this nursing home and to monitor
all nursing homes in the area.

Example 3: Staff members reported to the advocate a pattern of abuse in the dispensing of
narcotic drugs. Exploration revealed that one
or two doctors were issuing prescriptions care-
lessly, that pharmacists were in some instances
lax in filling prescriptions or reporting
abuses, and that several pharmacists were short-
changing on vital prescriptions because of what
they claimed were underpayments by Medicaid.
The advocate then reported this information to
the local enforcement agencies for action.

Example 4: Adverse reports reached the agency
about the local children's shelter: there was
indiscriminate mixing of all children regardless
of the reasons for being there, attendants were
neglectful, and some children were being victim-
ized by older children. Exploration indicated
that severe budget restrictions over the past
several years had resulted in understaffing,
poor morale, and inappropriate admissions. The
agency instigated investigations by several
county agencies, as well as gathering its own
documentation.

Relevance to Specific Client Groups

Although an agency, public or private, is providing a given service, that service may not be geared to the needs of certain groups in the community. The examples below illustrate the point. Often this problem stems from lack of understanding and staff training and can be remedied through action for staff inservice training.

Example 1: A local governmental agency had been trying to handle Hispanic applicants and clients by using as interpreters other Hispanics who happened to be in the waiting room. None of the staff members spoke or understood Spanish, and none of the literature or forms had Spanish equivalents. Exploration showed that the numbers of Hispanic people in the area had recently increased, and that the agency had not adapted to the new situation. Pressure from a group of agencies brought the problem to the attention of the agency's administration.

Example 2: A followup study of applicants and dropouts from an agency showed that women who had been raped and had made an initial contact had not returned. A check with other agencies disclosed similar experiences. The agency's advocate asked a women's group about the reasons. It appeared that the women felt not only that they had not been understood, but actually had been put down by the attitude of the counselors they encountered. The investigating agency proceeded to set up inservice training for its own staff and those of several other agencies.

Example 3: A board committee assessing needs in the area of criminal justice raised a question about the agency's service to the families of men with long-term prison sentences. An examination of the applications and caseload indicated that there were no actual cases, but there

had been several anonymous calls. Application
material showed that women had called but refused to give identifying data, and they seemed
"overly concerned" about confidentiality. Agency staff assigned to this advocacy project ex-
plored it extensively, finally learning that
this was an "invisible" group, very fearful and
ashamed, and needing a quite different reception
and treatment at agencies.

Planning Services for and with Clients

Another important area within local jurisdiction
of agencies, public and private, is the handling of
services at transition points. Many problems
arise: failure to follow up on clients; poor handling of transfer of clients to other facilities;
poor planning around discharge of people from a facility; failure to make any provision for those
whose application for service is rejected; and concern over dropouts from a service. Clients are often not planned with: they are given a plan or
perfunctorily asked to cooperate. Working through
of feelings is, of course, more time consuming but
is essential for the welfare of the client and may
well determine the outcome of the transition.

Example 1: Community and educational groups had
succeeded, after a long struggle, in getting several special schools established in the community for children with certain disabilities or
problems. Ironically, within a few years, a new
serious problem had arisen. The agency staff,
in working with families who had a child in one
of the special schools, found that no child ever
seemed to return to regular school, though the
purpose was to make this possible. Exploration
substantiated initial impressions. The regular
schools had no intention of taking back potentially troublesome children, nor did they follow
up on the children to determine their progress
and suitability for return to regular school.

With much effort the agency, together with parents and other groups, succeeded in getting the
school district to institute a careful followup
for annual evaluations of children in special
schools.

Example 2: Under a new mandate from Medicaid,
elderly patients in local nursing homes were re-
evaluated and many were judged to be fit for
other facilities. The agency soon began to hear
that patients were summarily moved - they were
told to pack up, taken to a vehicle, and trans-
ported to a new living situation, with no preparation. The agency, with other groups, immediately mounted a protest, resulting in adequate
preparation being built into the process. The
entire mechanism of reevaluation was called into
question through the courts.

Example 3: The agency received repeated complaints about inadequate discharge preparations
made for patients from a city hospital. Often
patients were turned out with no plan at all,
even when there were apparent health hazards.
The agency advocate asked hospital social workers what was happening and why no plans were
made; the workers claimed they were badly under-
staffed, and also that many patients were dis-
charged without the workers' knowledge. The
workers welcomed the agency's intervention to
remedy the situation.

Example 4: The agency became concerned over the
release of prisoners from the city jail after
several had walked into the agency, destitute,
homeless, and despondent. It was learned that
this was the common practice, and that the jail
authorities apparently felt they had no obligation to help prisoners plan for discharge. It
was found also that the jail staff made no effort to help families of prisoners, who often

asked for direction in regard to such matters as
financial difficulties and handling of children. An advocacy project was set up, aimed at
having jail staff trained to handle information
and referral needs on an elementary level, or
alternately to allow outside workers to enter to
help prisoners.

Example 5: Community concern over the practice
of a local treatment facility was taken up by
the agency. The facility rejected women applicants who could not get their husbands to come
with them initially for marital counseling, or
could not pay a fee based on their husband's income, despite the fact that the husband refused
to pay. Although it could not be determined
from the outside whether this was the facility's
policy or the practice of certain staff members,
a meeting with the administraion focused on an
interim plan of helping such rejected applicants
get help elsewhere, while the facility reconsid-
ered its position.

Example 6: The agency's advocacy committee, in
meeting with the local commissioner of social
services, became interested in the disposition
of those rejected for assistance. It appeared
that many who were only slightly over the eligibility level were indeed in desperate straits
and needed help even if the Department of Social
Service (DSS) could not assist them. A question
was then raised about referrals; it developed
that no planning was undertaken with those rejected. After further study, the committee
eventually proposed a plan to the DSS to ensure
that some form of help through referral was offered to everyone who applied.

Example 7: The advocate and board committee, in
studying their own agency experience in regard
to the referrals, came across several instances

of former clients who had been referred to a
training program and then dropped out of it.
Further exploration indicated that the training
facility did nothing in regard to dropouts, apparently assuming that other agencies would
somehow pick up on them. An advocacy action was
begun, aimed at having the facility provide inservice training for staff on this problem.

Administrative Problems

Included under this heading are a variety of
problems arising out of the administrative implementation of policies, laws, and regulations. The
usual results, from clients' points of view, are
lengthy delays or cutting off of benefits. The
problems generally are attributable to one or more
of such factors as cumbersome processing methods,
understaffing, rigid procedures, narrow interpretation of regulations and errors.

Example 1: Several clients going to a retrain-
ing facility complained that they lacked travel
money. The facility explained that they could
reimburse trainees only for actual expenses, and
that it took about six weeks for the first
claims to be processed by them and by the governmental office involved. The agency was able
to provide the small amounts needed, but took
this up as an advocacy cause, aiming to get the
procedures changed so that advances could be
made, rather than have the training program defeated.

Example 2: The agency received many reports of
lateness of voucher payments to vendors by the
local government, resulting in the refusal of
pharmacists to fill prescriptions, taxi drivers
to take clients, and other vendors to supply
medical equipment. The agency joined with many
others in bringing pressure to bear to change
this situation.

Example 3: Numerous clients complained that
they received checks late, especially when there
had been some change in status such as moving to
a new address or increase in size of family.
Investigation showed that the cause probably lay
in an inadequate computer system, and the agency, together with others, urged the local government to allocate funds to provide an up-to-
date computer service.

Example 4: An elderly couple, in poor health,
called the agency in a panic. They had received
word that they would receive no checks for three
months, because of overpayments in prior years.
They had already missed the first check. The
advocate found that both the local governmental
office and the federal were following a rigid
policy of immediate recoupment. Contacts with
officials produced a relaxation of the policy if
clients complained, so that only small amounts
were recouped at a time.

Example 5: An elderly widow appealed to the advocate to find out why she did not receive her
monthly check; she was unable to get out to a
pay phone to make the repeated calls necessary.
The advocate uncovered a bizarre situation - the
computer had rejected her card on the grounds
that she was dead. Weeks were lost in trying to
determine what had gone wrong and in trying to
produce the documentation that would pass the
computer. Although it proved impossible to
trace what apparently was a computer error, she
was finally reestablished in her benefits.

Example 6: The advocate received reports from
staff working with the elderly that clients were
required to appear with their birth certificates
for recertification at the government office.
This was quite a hardship for many who were in
poor health or disabled, and who found both the

trip and the day-long wait at the office difficult and exhausting. Meeting with the supervisors of the government office, the advocate
pointed out that since they already had copies
of the birth certificates on file, it was hardly
necessary to have them copied each time - and
that proof of age of 65 or older was also unnecessary, since the clients obviously did not get
younger! The officials agreed finally to at
least waive the visit on request, and to handle
recertifications by mail.

Example 7: In one area, a governmental office
had arranged to deposit checks directly into
clients' bank accounts to prevent theft from
mail boxes, and to relieve elderly or disabled
clients from having to cash the checks, with
possible danger of the theft of cash. Several
clients complained to the agency, however, that
they had run into trouble. They had written
checks to pay rent and utilities against their
account, only to find the checks had bounced.
Due to some error, their checks had not been de-
posited. The advocate learned that the governmental office had no provision for notifying a
client of the deposit, and the bank did so only
at monthly intervals. The advocate pointed out
that while the regulations did not specify notification to the client - and so it had not been
done - such notification was not prohibited.
Officials agreed to consider how they could make
this change in what was otherwise a very helpful
procedure.

Publicizing of Services; Outreach

There are many difficulties in bringing to people's attention helpful benefits, entitlements, and
services. Often the publicity does not reach those
groups who most need the benefits. Announcements
in the newspapers hardly suffice, and a much broader effort is needed. While the obligation is

heavier upon governmental offices, private agencies also should make known what they have to offer in this connection.

Example 1: An agency serving a large area of both urban and rural communities found that clients were not aware of their eligibility for food stamps. On contacting the local food stamp office, the staff found that far less than 50 percent of the eligible people had applied. The action undertaken aimed both at increased publicity by all organizations and at the employment of outreach workers by the government office.

Example 2: The agency learned that many of the elderly in the community did not know of benefits, discounts, and opportunities provided through the local government. The advocate was told by the government office that there had been frequent newspaper publicity. It was suggested that the office issue a brochure covering all the provisions and distribute it widely through home delivery, supermarkets, and pharmacies.

Example 3: Although the local government had become eligible to provide rent subsidies, the announcement was not clear and it appeared that many persons were not eligible. The advocate learned that the city office was still confused about the eligibility requirements. The advocate pressed to have clarification obtained quickly, with further publicity, not only in the newpapers, but also to agencies and community organizations.

Example 4: The agency found that clients on welfare usually were unaware of rights or opportunities available to them. Many could not understand printed material given to them because of its legalistic language. The agency assigned

staff to work with a clients' group and other
organizations on a manual for welfare clients,
explaining in everyday language their rights,
opportunities, and the actual steps required
with the welfare offices.

Enforcement

Problems develop often through lack of enforcement of laws or failure to carry out services. In
some instances they may mean that there are powerful forces operating against enforcement and that
change will not be easy; in other situations, it
may result from ingrained attitudes and practices.
Advocacy may attempt directly to obtain enforcement
or focus on other measures that may have the same
result.

Example 1: Outreach workers of an agency found
that tenants in several adjoining buildings were
suffering from gross failure on the landlord's
part to make necessary repairs. The advocate
and the outreach workers obtained full documentation of the problem from a group of the tenants. To the advocate's surprise, however, the
tenants begged him not to contact the local government for enforcement of the building codes
and health regulations because the landlord
would evict them and, with the housing shortage,
they might be worse off. The advocate then ex-
plored other possibilities, such as a rent
strike, which the tenants again opposed. Finally, the advocate, working with other agencies
and the local government, developed a housing
relocation service that would find other places
for tenants if any were evicted. With this in
hand, the advocate finally met with the landlord, who agreed to make at least some repairs
rather than have the buildings shut down.

Example 2: The agency, learning of reports from
other parts of the country of stores over-

charging residents of low-income areas, sent out several volunteer advocate/investigators, who continued the reports. Drug stores, for example, regularly charged much more than in other parts of the city, and chain stores and supermarkets often failed to have the same sales or discounts. Agency staff contacted the local governmental officials responsible to determine what powers of enforcement they had and whether they were willing to take action.

Example 3: Residents of a low-income, predominantly minority area complained to outreach workers that there was little, if any, police protection for the area, and that the more that conditions worsened, the more the police stayed away. Agency staff met informally with police officials, then with policemen assigned to the area. It was learned that the policemen saw the area as hostile, with residents presenting the appearance of the police; signs of racial discrimination were also evident. The agency discussed with officials the possibility of the department's providing much more training, including special help on handling of family violence and on ways of working with a community. The agency proposed a joint project with the department in which agency staff would cooperate with the police on specific situations that arose; the outreach workers, who were for the most part residents of the area, would play a key role in the shaping and execution of the plan.

Example 4: Agency clients who visited their children in a nearby summer camp complained to their caseworkers about conditions at the camp - lack of safety provisions and poor food, for example. The people who ran the camp brushed off their concerns. The advocate visited the camp but was also rebuffed. The parents, working with the advocate, filed formal complaints with county officials and maintained pressure on the officials to enforce safety, food, and health regulations.

LACK OF SERVICES

While ineffective service is a major cause for many local problems, there is a second cause that is so obvious that its significance may be over-looked. Community problems and needs frequently exist because there are no services to respond to them. Sometimes, these services can be obtained only through broader action - through state or federal legislation. Yet there are many that can be established through local efforts. Sometimes an agency can fill a need by broadening the scope of an existing service. On the other hand, the population group needing the service may want to organize a new agency. Usually, local conditions determine the path to be followed, depending on the need, the resources, community attitudes, and the flexibility of existing agencies.

Many kinds of local problems offer the possibility of advocacy action. The accompanying checklist identifies nineteen problem areas and suggests services that may be needed to help in each area. An agency, reviewing the list, will discover opportunities for advocacy in its community when it sees the number of services that are presently lacking.

CHECKLIST OF SERVICES[1]
1. Food and clothing
   Emergency food and clothing provisions
   Free or subsidized meals, at sites, in homes, in and out of school programs for children
   Clothing provision - free or subsidized, uniform and work supplies
2. Housing
   Shelter for homeless, transients, etc.
   Housing counseling, information, location assistance

Rehabilitation, repair, renovation, restoration, etc.
Mortgage and loan assistance
Provision of furniture, supplies, tools, etc.
Public housing
Rent subsidy
Retirement housing, centers, communities
Urban homestead
Building, housing code enforcement, fair housing, land use
3. Financial resources
Emergency financial assistance
Financial counseling
AFDC
General financial assistance
Food stamps
Social security
Supplemental Security Income
Unemployment insurance
Veterans' benefits
Workman's compensation
Other disability, retirement, death benefits
Health insurance - including Medicare, Medicaid
4. Employment
Counseling, testing
Job development
Training - on the job, public service, etc.
Sheltered employment
Job placement
Assistance to handicapped groups
Homebound employment
Enforcement of equal opportunity, affirmative action, minimum wage, etc.
5. Education
Educational counseling, information
Diagnostic evaluation
Schools - preschool through high school
Special education - disabled, emotional and behavior problems, gifted, developmentally disabled, handicapped, learning disorders, etc.
Vocational education

Colleges, graduate schools
Technical schools
Tutoring
Provision of textbooks
Equal educational opportunity
Homebound instruction
Continuing and adult education
6. Health
Counseling, information
Emergency medical care
Testing, diagnostic evaluation
Home health care
General medical care - outpatient
Medical care - inpatient
Dental care
Infant stimulation
Alternative care - nursing homes, family care,
intermediate facility, etc.
Rehabilitation
Blood banks
Provision of medication, medical supplies and
equipment
Screening, and prevention
Health reporting and statistics
7. Recreation and cultural
Activity groups - adults, children, youth, aged
Arts appreciation
Camping - residential, day
Libraries
Lectures, discussions, exhibitions, etc.
Special rates for groups
Special programs - Handicapped, developmentally
disabled, etc.
8. Social-emotional development, adjustment
Emergency services - drug, alcohol, mental
health, etc.
Personal and family counseling - including
special groups such as aged, alcoholics,
children, homosexuals, physically handicapped,
drug abusers, etc.
Diagnostic and evaluative services

Hospitalization, partial hospitalization
Self-help groups
Social interaction groups
Reassurance service
Companionship service - including foster
grandparents, Big Brother, etc.

9. <u>Protection from abuse, neglect, exploitation</u>
Education, information service
Protective services - adults, children
Shelter
Investigation services - adults, children

10. <u>Assistance in homemaking</u>
Chore services
Homemaker services
Educational services
Assistance to aged, disabled

11. <u>Day care</u>
After-school care
Education and information
Centers - including for developmentally
disabled, elderly, emotionally disturbed,
handicapped
Family day care

12. <u>Family planning</u>
Counseling and information
Pregnancy counseling and information
Sexual functioning - counseling and information

13. <u>Adoption</u>
Counseling and information
Evaluation
Placement
Supervision
Guidance

14. <u>Substitute living arrangements</u>
Emergency shelter care - adults, children,
special groups (drug, alcohol, youth, etc.)
Foster family care - children, aged,
delinquents, etc.
Group homes - for various groups
Residential care
Residential treatment care

Transitional services - halfway houses, etc.
Counseling, information
Placement
15. Consumer Protection
Regulation of business practices
Weights and measures
Information services
Safety standards
Buying groups
16. Environment - protection, safety, enrichment
Sanitation, etc.
Beautification, preservation
Traffic
Environmental health inspection
Control of hazards, pests, etc.
Water supply
Pollution abatement
Regulation and licensing of day care, foster
homes, residential facilities, etc.
17. Community safety and justice
Fire prevention, control, protection
Crime prevention and protection
Law enforcement, police
Court services
Legal defense services
Civil liberties organizations
Probation, parole
Detention facilities
Services for offenders, ex-offenders
Delinquency prevention services
Pre-trial services
Disaster relief
Civil defense
Weather warnings
Land/water rescue
Rape victims counseling, information
Consumer safety
18. Community organization and information
Information dissemination and referral
Information and referral service
Community education and information (on alcohol,

consumer affairs, drugs, environmental problems,
mental health, health, etc.)
Advocacy (generally and in relation to various
subjects - child care, education, consumers,
housing, legal issues, etc.)
Charitable foundations
Voluntary fund raising
Community and human relations
Civil rights
Community planning
Neighborhood development
Economic development (small business, industry,
tourism, etc.)
Occupational and professional groups
Political parties
Service planning
Volunteers (recruitment, placement, training,
types of uses, etc.)
19. Transportation
Car pool information
Transportation information
Emergency medical transportation
Errand-running service
Escort services
Public transit
Reduced rates
Special transit (for disabled, aged, school
children, etc.)

The following examples illustrate some of the
categories of services in the checklist, showing
needs for services and the ways in which agencies
became aware of them. The numbers in parentheses
following each example refer to the category in the
checklist.

Advocacy problems often embrace a cluster of
needs for service rather than a single need. Thus,
the problem of battered women may point up such
needs as emergency shelter, housing, counseling,
and legal defense.

Example 1:   The agency, becoming aware of increasing emergency needs in the community due to
unemployment and cuts in public assistance,
called together concerned organizations to coordinate voluntary help for emergency food, clothing, and shelter. (1 and 2)

Example 2: Project staff in a neighborhood center reported to the agency director that many of
the minority youths with whom they worked were
blocked by the lack of employment, whether they
were in school or out. The board-staff committee set up to study the problem found that there
was no employment service focusing on the particular needs of youth. The committee asked the
director to recommend to the council of agencies
(which included the head of the local office of
the State Employment Service) that priority be
given to development of such service. (4)

Example 3: Caseworkers in the agency, knowing
about problems encountered by children of families in counseling, reported to the advocate
that the local school system did not seem to
have any provision for children with learning
disabilities. The advocate launched a study and
was finally able to obtain definite information
that the school lacked any specific helping
methods for such children. An advocacy action
was then set in motion, involving other agencies
and groups, to press for special educational arrangements. (5)

Example 4: The agency received several applications from women for emergency help with rent,
food, and other necessities. Outreach workers
visiting the women found that a crisis had been
precipitated when the husbands had been senten-
ced to prison; wives and children were suddenly
left without means and didn't know what to do.
They were also ashamed and fearful of revealing

their plight. The outreach workers pointed out that, based on the numbers sent to prison annually from the community, there were many women and children in a similar position; a specialized reach-out service was needed. (8)

Example 5: At a meeting of an agency advisory committee made up of senior citizens, staff learned that one of the most stressful problems encountered by seniors in the community was that of repair of small appliances and minor house repairs. Many of the senior citizens owned their own houses, but fixed low incomes precluded their paying for such work. Many also were unable to take care of other essential tasks, such as putting up storm windows and screens, and clearing away snow. The advocate assigned a graduate student to visit homes in one neighborhood to determine the prevalence of the problems and provide a basis for developing a service. (10)

Example 6: Agency staff, through frequent contacts with the school social workers, became aware that the school system glossed over problems of pregnant girls. The school social workers believed that an outside agency might have more influence than they had had. The agency found that several interrelated services were needed: counseling, health education, health care, and continuance of education. An action plan to obtain the needed services was developed and presented to school officials.

Example 7: The agency director received word that funds for the local legal service for low-income people had been drastically cut, along with several other services. He learned, after further calls, that a sudden decision had been made at a state level due to shifts in federal funding. Working with a board committee, the director joined in action with other agencies throughout the state, but it was decided that this would be a lengthy process and that a serious gap in service had to be remedied, if only temporarily. Staff were finding that already many low-income clients had to be turned away from the legal service. The advocate developed a plan to recruit volunteer lawyers and to involve the local bar association in developing further supplementary help. (17)

Example 8: A study of agency statistics over a five-year period showed a large increase in information calls from people living in new suburban areas and in rural areas in two counties adjacent to the city. Discussion with staff, including receptionists, brought out that callers often complained about getting the runaround, about not knowing where to call, or not finding anyone who knew where they should call. The directory used by staff proved to be not only outdated but incomplete, especially in regard to the counties involved. A board-staff advocacy committee found that the county Departments of Social Service had not carried out a mandate to establish information and referral services. It was decided to press for action by the public agencies by forming a coalition of private agencies to work with the public agencies, which had funding available to them. (18)

For the sake of clarity, this chapter has discussed the advocacy issues in local problems from two perspectives - problems that exist because of ineffective services and problems that exist because of lack of services. The distinction, in reality, is not always easy to make and is useful only to provide reference points for the start of advocacy initiatives.

5

METHOD: THE STUDY

Advocacy is still in an early stage of development in many agencies. It is a process that can be
conceptualized simply and clearly as having four
major divisions. Persons familiar with social
casework will see a similarity in concept: casework
can be divided into diagnosis, treatment plan,
treatment, and evaluation, while advocacy has similar divisions - study, planning, action, and evaluation.

Advocacy does not yet rest on any extensive body
of knowledge derived from research. It operates on
practice knowledge constructed from assembling experiences. In contrast, casework has slowly developed a body of research though it also depends
heavily on experience. Research in casework is not
without problems and advocacy research, as it
grows, will encounter similar, if not more difficult, issues.

The process of advocacy is similar to casework
process from another viewpoint. In casework, the
initial interview marks the beginning of treatment,
though in the conceptual framework the process involves diagnosis, plan, and then treatment. In a
comparable way, in advocacy, action may occur at
the beginning of the process. Thus the conceptual
framework seems artificial and awkward, especially
to practitioners. But its value is in helping the

organizing of experience and knowledge so that the practitioner gains skill in using it effectively.

In theory about social change, there is much research on innovation, the spreading of change.[1] At first glance, this activity would seem to be pertinent to advocacy, but the focus of the research is peripheral and it cannot be used directly in the advocacy process. This research on innovation, as well as research on organization behavior, has been developed into certain principles in Jack Rothman's Planning and Organizing for Social Change. In a subsequent volume, Promoting Innovation and Change in Organizations and Communities, Rothman, John L. Erlich, and Joseph G. Teresa describe the application of several principles to social work process. To this extent, the research can be helpful in limited aspects of the study and planning phases of the advocacy process.

To make another distinction, advocacy and community organization are not synonymous. Advocacy may be differentiated from community organization when the latter is defined as a planning and coordinating function. For example, the lack of coordination among public and private services might be the target of an advocacy action; at the point where there is agreement on a remedy, community organization skills would be used to work out the actual coordination.

Advocacy is perhaps characterized most clearly, in this comparison, by its adversarial stance directed against defects or lacks in existing systems, against target institutions that resist change. In recent years, efforts have been made to incorporate the advocacy stance into the overall concept of community organization, principally by adding "conflictual" activities to the "consensus" type usually associated with community organization.[2] It would seem clearer, however, and more related to practice, to consider advocacy as a separate method, with its own concepts, framework, and intervention techniques.

THE STUDY

The study phase of the advocacy process is presented in this chapter as a single, separate unit. In practice, some elements of the study may have been done during the process of selecting the given problem from among other possible issues for advocacy. The need for some information may be uncovered during the planning phase, and still other information may be obtained during the action - for example, an action may start off with a survey, with the results then being fed back into the study and the planning.

Though there is interplay between the phases of the advocacy process, much of the study must be carried out systematically near the beginning of the process to form a solid basis for planning. For example, in one action it was assumed that a local government office had decision-making powers; after considerable activity, the advocacy delegation met with the officials only to be told that the state government had to make the decision. The entire advocacy process had to be reoriented.

On occasion part of the advocacy action has to be directed at obtaining information from an organization that resists giving it. The advocates will have to proceed without all the information needed, establishing the preliminary goal of obtaining the information.

This chapter is divided into four parts: problem, target organization or system, advocate organization and supporting groups, and proposed change.

The Problem

It is assumed here that the process of selecting and defining the problem or issue has already taken place, but it is helpful to start the study with an initial restatement of the problem, in specific terms and without mixing in goals or methods. This sets a base for the study and avoids prejudging possible solutions.

For example, the original definition might be: "To form a coalition to pressure the state legislature into providing funds for services to battered women and their children." This type of statement does not state the problem; it spells out the conclusions of a study and a plan, and there may be other solutions more feasible than having a new law passed, with funding. A coalition might not be useful or, even more likely, might be but one of several major thrusts. A restatement of the problem in the following way - "There is a lack of specific services such as an emergency residence, counseling, legal services for battered women" - gives guidance in developing the study.

The statement of the problem obviously is not definitive since, as a result of the study, the problem may be refocused or broadened.

The study requires information about the source of knowledge of the problem. Did the agency learn of it through clients (case to cause)? Or through outside information that the problem existed (public issue)? A written statement about the source is important so that others who become involved in the advocacy effort can be clear about it. Where possible, clients should be brought into the study and planning phases; or, if it is a public issue, one of the first steps may be to seek out some of those affected by the problem. This requires a separate planning and action phase.

Three other questions are important at this stage: who is affected by the problem, what are

the consequences of the problem, and what is its
history?

Who is affected? Some estimate of the number of
people already affected, or who will definitely
be affected, is useful. A range of figures or,
depending on the problem, some data from which
estimates can be deduced, may be obtainable.
Other demographic data should also be sought:
for example, ages, geographical locations, income levels, ethnicity, cultural group, unemployment, educational level. Sources of information include census data, with detailed break-
down by tracts or lesser units; planning commis-
sions; utility companies; business associations;
surveys; interviews with selected individuals;
newspaper files; local publications. Other organizations may have made studies in the past
that are still useful.

What are the consequences? The study should determine the urgency. Is there a time deadline?
Are the consequences so drastic that quick action is called for? The severity of the problem
has to do with its effect upon people. Are basic needs involved - food, shelter, safety? More
complex needs - family relationships, well-
being, psychological health, neighborhood morale, and human rights and dignity? Indirect results are also important, as well as the future
implications if the problem continues. It is
useful to estimate social cost, especially for
use in publicity when costs can be documented as
resulting from the problem.

What is the history? Information is needed on
how the problem arose. Many problems can be
traced to a specific data, to a ruling or law or
event; others may be chronic conditions that
have gradually worsened or become more notice-
able. The study should explore the forces or

factors that gave rise to the problem, and whether they or others are maintaining the problem. This aspect ties into the study of the target organization or system. It is also helpful to determine why the problem has surfaced now, and whether this has meaning for the development of the advocacy plan and action.

History also includes prior efforts, if any, to tackle the problem - who tried, what methods were used, what was the outcome? - as well as current efforts to ameliorate it. This information can help advocates avoid past mistakes or identify external factors that promise more favorable conditions.

The study should also explore possible interested groups and organizations, and gather names of individuals who might lend support.

Target Organization or System

Problems of the kind that advocacy programs deal with are usually located in an organization or system of organizations, and it is possible to pinpoint the specific organization in which the problem occurs. This would not be true of such a problem as adverse attitudes prevalent in a community toward a particular ethnic group. However, advocacy tends to be directed toward organizations that have a human service product - units of government at various levels, private organizations, and sometimes business organizations.

Organizational behavior has been widely studied. Jack Rothman has written, "Unlike other practice issue areas, organizational research has a definite tradition of theory and research development representing a coherent school of scholarly endeavor...Because of the cognitive and philosophical orientation of the researchers, most of the studies lend themselves to application in terms of administrative and planning issues, rather than social action."[3] There are, nevertheless, some principles drawn from organizational research that are relevant to advocacy; also, an understanding of organizational behavior will give the advocate and those associated in advocacy efforts an understanding of organizations useful in developing advocacy strategy.

With human life so intertwined with organizational life, an understanding of the complexity of linkages among organizations is important in any advocacy effort. Organizations are combined into coalitions, federations, councils, congresses, and chambers.[4]

Organizational theory early focused on bureaucracy, with Weber originally seeing it as the best model for the rational organization of complex activity, and later emphasizing its shortcomings in practice.[5] Two major subsequent approaches drew on behavioral theory and systems theory.[6] In the latter approach, the organization was analyzed as an open system, depending upon such elements as inputs, outputs, and feedback, a useful way of conceptualizing an organization for study in an advocacy effort.

Three of the main organization processes are particularly relevant for advocacy:
1) Decision-making process. Decision making is composed of dynamically related steps, however differently labelled by various authors. One source, for example, identifies them as the problem, the identification of the objectives, the identification of alternative solutions, the evaluations of alternatives, the choice.[7] In broad terms, decision making in management is the same as the problem-solving steps outlined for the advocacy process.

2) <u>Organizational communications</u>. Studies of communication problems and methods are of interest, especially in relation to upward and horizontal communication methods.[8] Information theory, originated in the 1940s by Norbert Weiner and Claude Shannon, deals with the mathematical and transmission aspects of communications. Communication techniques involve such relatively familiar features as grievance procedure, open-door policy by superiors, counseling, attitude questionnaires, exit interviews, and participation methods for decision making.

3) <u>Control</u>. This refers to the functions usually labeled in social work as "accountability," "evaluation," "review," and "monitoring." It is aimed at answering the question, how did the activity turn out, or how is it going? The systems approach is useful here, in the concept of feedback, built into operations in order to give an ongoing picture of the status of an activity.

General systems theory, developed during the 1950s, has been widely applied. A system is defined as "a set of interacting parts contained within a boundary."[9] Other definitions are similar, emphasizing the interacion and interdependence of parts, and the interchanges with the environment (other systems, in effect). A number of familiar terms are associated with the theory - feedback, monitoring, tradeoffs, interfaces, entropy, coping, adaptation. Efforts have been made to incorporate this approach into social work, starting in the late 1960s.[10]

The ecosystem, a special system within general systems theory, is concerned with the adaptations and relations between living organisms and their environments. In social work, the ecological approach refers to this special system in relation to human beings and their institutions. The adaptive processes involve such activity as coping, changing the environment and self, and interfacing between systems. These ideas parallel those of Heinz Hartmann, who developed the conception of the ego as an adaptive organ "...utilizing the alloplastic or autoplastic maneuvers" - changing the environment or changing the self toward better adaptation.[11]

For advocacy, the systems approach has already enhanced understanding of human organizations and, it is hoped, will eventually lead to the specificity needed for practical advocacy actions. Thus far, the systems approach has provided the linkage between the field of organizational functioning and behavior and the field of individual interactions with the organizational environment.

A system of organizations is exemplified, for our purpose, by the welfare system of the local, state, and federal agencies administering welfare. Note, however, that each such agency can belong to other systems as well - the local department of social services belongs to the city government, for example.

When advocacy is directed toward unmet needs rather than toward malfunctions in organizations, the identity of the target organization or system may not be immediately clear. In the statement of an advocacy problem such as "There is a need for an emergency shelter for battered women," no target organization is specified. With study, one or more target organizations may be identified as potential initiators of a needed service.

Once a target organization or system has been pinpointed, certain information about the organization is necessary to design strategy: legal basis, relationship to community, goals, formal and

informal power structure, decision makers, reaction
to criticism, and supportive or allied organizations.

Legal basis. Probably most of the target organizations with which advocacy deals have a legal
basis for their activities, as differentiated
from social groups or other informal associations of people. Units of local government are
legally based in the local government, though
the latter often is acting under a delegation of
authority from a higher level of government.
Some local units may be created by the state, or
the local government may have the option to
adopt them. Private organizations are usually
incorporated or chartered under state law; this
may be of some importance if the question is
raised whether the organization is violating its
charter or, in the case of a public unit, ex-
ceeding its authority.

It is important also to determine whether
there are superordinates - higher level organizations exercising some degree of control over
the target organization. Thus, an organization
chartered by the state may be violating local
health requirements, and be subject to action by
the Department of Health. Or, a mental health
clinic, chartered as an independent organization
with its own board of directors, may be subject
to state licensing requirements and, if it re-
ceives funds from the local government, may also
be subject to various local regulations and requirements. Some governmental units are part of
a clear superordinate structure: the local Social Security office, for example, is a unit in
a structure culminating directly in the Social
Security Administration on the federal level.

The legal basis of a private nonprofit organization usually provides for the basic struc-

tural elements: officers of the corporation and the board of directors, and an executive to whom authority is delegated and who in turn directs staff. If incorporated as a membership organization, the body of members elects the board of directors. In public units, elected officials command a structure of department heads or similar subdivisions. It is important to know the way in which the structure below the board or official level is determined.

Relationship to community. One aspect of relationship to the community is the extent to which the target organization is involved with other organizations in councils, in working relationships, and in joint projects. Information should be obtained on all of these since they represent possible sources of influence on the target organization. Another aspect is the extent to which the community is involved in the conduct of the organization. How is the board of directors of a private nonprofit organization made up? Are citizens or consumers involved in any way with the conduct of a governmental unit? Does the target organization have any formal ways of eliciting community response, such as public hearings? Does the organization issue documents such as reports and brochures? Does it have formal mechanisms for individual complaints, appeals, or information seeking? At what levels within the organization do interchanges with the community take place, apart from the direct service rendered?

Goals. While an organization's goals may be originally stated in its incorporation documents or enabling legislation, these original statements have usually been modified and adapted by practice over time, though within the general meaning of the original goals. Most organizations have goal statements, that is, statements of what they are trying to do. These should be examined to determine whether its activities seem consonant with the stated goals, or whether in practice the organization has significantly deviated from them. This information can later be used in various ways: in publicity it may be pointed out that the organization is falling far short of its goals, or seems to be going against them; other bodies, such as advisory committees, may bring their influence to bear upon an organization, if they believe there are serious discrepancies.

Goals may be expressed in various ways. One pattern includes official goals and operating goals. Another distinguishes product goals from internal goals. There are system goals and societal goals.[12]

Two types of goals may be of particular significance in advocacy: maintenance and legitimization. The former refers to the goal of maintaining the organization, specifically the resources the organization requires to continue, and the internal dynamics and structure than keep it functioning. This suggests on the one hand that threats to the survival of an organization are likely to meet with intense opposition and, on the other hand, pressure brought to bear on the source of support of the organization may influence change.

Legitimization refers to the need of the organization for public approval. Sometimes, determining what part or level of an organization is more sensitive to public opinion will help to make advocacy efforts more effective.

Finally, rewording of goals by an organization may reveal some kind of a response to the public. For example, the change from "Depart-

ment of Welfare" to "Department of Social Services" is in effect a new goal statement, though
nothing else may have changed at that point.
New expectations are set up by the new wording,
affecting evaluation of its work and personnel.

Formal and informal power structures. In addition to the top-level power structure - officers, directors, chief executive - large organizations have lower strata, formal delegations of
power to heads of subdivisions and below them to
lower management positions. Other small, separate subdivisions may have formalized power and
report directly to top-level management. For
example, in a large department of social services, headed by a commissioner and two deputy
commissioners who direct major subsidivions,
there are also a small legal divison and a small
controller's division, each of which exercises
veto power over operations and interrelates on
this basis with major subsidivisions.

An ongoing advocacy program may soon develop
a working knowledge of the major target organizations and their formal power structure, but it
is necessary to keep updating this information,
due to frequent reorganizations occurring in
large organizations.

Informal power alignments are not discernible
through charts or literature of the target organizations. Reports from within the target organizations and experiences of staff and others
in contact with the target organization form the
basis for understanding the informal system.[13]
Informal power stems from such factors as the
personal abilities of an individual or his or
her outside connections - political clout or
connections to influential board members, for
example. Thus, of three individuals at the same
level, one may have more real power than the

other two, and may overshadow an immediate superior; higher level management may rely on this person's opinions.

Power struggles go on in most large organizations, at times intensely, revolving around turf struggles between one part of an organization and another, or around the efforts of an individual to advance by displacing someone above.

The advocate needs to know as much as possible of the informal power alignments and struggles, either to use them to advantage or to avoid having the issue become caught up in internal conflicts and consequently blocked or defeated.

Decision makers. It is important to identify at which level in a large organization a decision for change can be made, or at what level a favorable recommendation to a chief executive will be effective. Often this may not be clear, even to those on the inside, and a person who thinks he or she can make a decision has to back down and refer the matter on. On the other hand, it may be unwise to bother a top-level management person with a matter than can be settled at a lower level, especially if pressure is brought to enable the advocate to reach the chief executive on the matter. Settling issues at a lower level is important when the strategy is to keep the conflictual level low in order to resolve it informally and without public visibility. The development of too much outside pressure will tend to raise the conflictual level, polarize the issue, and produce unnecessary resistance. When this happens, the advocacy effort is out of control.

Reaction to criticism. Organizations will vary in their responses to public criticism, depend-

ing on such factors as the style of the top-
level people and the current political climate.
Over time, an advocate can become familiar with
the typical stances of organizations. Some may
take conciliatory positions publicly, which may
or may not indicate any real willingness to
change. Others may typically counterattack.
Still others may respond more subtly through
promotional efforts that indirectly answer, min-
imize, or otherwise dismiss criticism. Knowing
these characteristics helps the advocate's strategy: it may be fruitless to mount a publicity
campaign against an organization that typically
is unresponsive to outside criticism, unless
there is reason to think it has recently developed a vulnerability.

Supportive or allied organizations. Knowing
whether a target organization belongs to coherent systems from which is draws support is important. Thus, a unit of local government usually will be supported by local government, at
least publicly, and possibly by state government
or by the dominant political party; these usually have a strong investment in the target organization. In contrast, a private nonprofit organization may be loosely allied with similar
organizations, which do not have any specific
investment and may rather easily withdraw support. Also, some community groups will tend to
rally to the target organization, just as there
are others that may side with the advocate
group.

Potential supporting groups of a target organization should be studied sufficiently to understand what the ties are and what counterin-
terests such groups may have that would weaken
their support. For example, certain groups tend
to support restrictive welfare policies of a local department of social services, yet their

support may not be forthcoming if the issue is focused on waste of taxpayers' money by the department.

Research shows, however, that it is usually not profitable to attempt to influence diehard groups, as it requires great expenditure of effort with very uncertain results.[14]

Vulnerabilities of target organizations. The purpose of the study of the target organization is primarily to indicate in what ways the decision makers can be reached under conditions favoring the desired resolution of the issue. The clearer and more complete this part of the study is, the easier is the task in planning or selecting appropriate intervention techniques and of setting the overall strategy. Some research in organizational behavior bears indirectly on vulnerabilities. (Jack Rothman has provided examples of action guidelines deduced from research studies.[15]) The study cannot provide exact measurements and invariable conditions regarding the target organization, and the information available can serve only as a guide, but this is obviously more helpful than relying upon scattered, unrelated bits of information. The advocate and the planning group will have a greater chance of success if the study is adequately developed.

Advocate Organization and Supporting Groups

Although it may seem unnecessary for the staff and board of an advocate agency to have an available study of their own agency, outsiders who become involved in the advocacy effort will probably have only a vague idea of the agency as an organization, with its strengths and weaknesses. Thus, formalized information on the agency's goals, structure, and operations should be prepared. In relation to a given advocacy action, it is also

helpful to have an assessment of possible constraints on agency action, from within and without
the agency. This is particularly important for
client groups; otherwise they may, because of their
plight, tend to overvalue the agency's power and
have unrealistic expectations. Or the clients may
lack confidence in the agency's capacity to help
them, and their lack of understanding of the agency
may increase anxiety and distrust.

The resources potentially available for advocacy
in an agency have already been described in chapter
2. Theoretical material on participation in advocacy can be found in Rothman.[16] Some of the action
guidelines on participation developed by Rothman
from the research studies were put into operation
and studied in Promoting Innovation and Change in
Organizations and Communities.[17]

Proposed Change

This phase of the study of the problem is an examination of alternative ways of resolving it and
it may lead to restatement of the problem. While a
problem may seem to have only one resolution, other
possible solutions should be posed. For example,
an emergency shelter for battered women may appear
to be the only solution, yet local factors such as
funding difficulties may make this highly unlikely. If the problem is restated to indicate the
need rather than the solution, then other possibilities can emerge - foster homes in the community,
use of motels, for example.

Creative thinking is particularly important when
the advocacy action is directed toward unmet
needs. Traditional solutions that come readily to
mind may not be the best solutions. Also, innovative approaches often help the advocacy action succeed, because of greater appeal or lower cost or
other favorable elements. Innovative approaches
can be developed by checking the literature on what

has been tried elsewhere. Or creative thinking may be stimulated by examining aspects of a solution: delivery methods, operational methods, types of personnel - speculating on how each might be varied from the usual solution. Clients, from their special perspective, may be able to point out neglected approaches.

Possible constraints in proposed solutions should be examined, such as high cost, specialized personnel, or inappropriateness to the community or client group. Also important is the way in which the proposed solution fits in with the target organization's overall pattern of operating. Rogers, in Diffusion of Innovations, points out that innovations are more likely to be adopted if they are generally congruent with the organization's existing goals, structure, and methods, rather than being startling departures. Successful demonstration projects, for example, often fail to be taken up on a broad scale because they have been developed outside existing systems and vary too greatly from the system's norms.

The study of alternatives also provides the opportunity during the planning and action phase for accepting compromise solutions.

6

METHOD: PLANNING

Clear and specific goals should be set down for
each advocacy plan. Otherwise, the action becomes
diffuse, unlikely to arrive at any outcome, and unable to provide accountability. Thus, an advocacy
goal "to press for national health insurance" provides no guide to action, and the only measure
would be the final achievement of national health
insurance, hardly a likely outcome of a small-scale
effort. A more realistic goal, to the same end,
would be "to increase public awareness of the need
for national health insurance through a community
education program including public meetings, media
coverage, and special literature."

In practice, a preliminary formulation of goals
should be made, and then at the end of the planning
process, a final statement should be articulated.
The preliminary statement serves as a guide to the
plan - the strategy and intervention techniques -
which in turn often leads to a better formulation
of the goals as capabilities and resources are
matched against possibilities.

GOALS

Each advocacy plan should involve consideration
of three types of goals:
The problem goal. This should specify the
change sought within the given target organization or system, with enough clarity that

outcomes can be compared to goals. Example: To have the city government rescind the budget cuts in the home health aide program.

Participation goal. This should elaborate the groups and kinds of individuals, inside and outside the agency, to be involved in the advocacy action, and the goals in terms of the values to be achieved by the participants. Example: To include in the advocacy action regarding budget cuts a board committee, staff, a group of senior citizen clients of the agency, the Council of Senior Citizen Clubs, and the local chapter of the American Association of Retired Persons; the purpose is to help senior groups gain some empowerment and overcome feelings of helplessness and apathy, to enhance their sense of common purposes, and to help board members understand more directly the plight of the elderly and their need for help in acting in their own behalf.

Education goal. This refers to making an educational impact upon the broader community. Efforts may be diffused through mass media or focused upon particular areas or groups. Example: To increase the community's awareness of the plight of the elderly and the need for supports to maintain them in the community, and to reach as many senior citizens as possible in the community to enlist their support for this and other causes.

Most advocacy actions lend themselves to all three goals, and, at the minimum, all three should be considered for each advocacy plan. Because of its action orientation, advocacy focuses most upon the problem; but the other two goals will broaden and enrich the plans.

Also, advocacy is more than a series of discrete actions. It is an ongoing thrust and movement in behalf of a cause, and each action fits into and contributes to the advancing of that cause. Advocacy is incremental, building support and understanding continually.

Focusing only on the problem results in measuring outcome only in terms of success or failure in solving the problem. This can lead to plans that seem most likely to settle the problem, but at the expense of the other goals. For example, several members of the advocate agency board have strong influence on the city mayor and believe they can resolve the problem quickly through an informal, unpublicized meeting; this would mean that other people concerned could not be brought into the action.

Such a situation poses difficult value judgments for the agency: Would a broader advocacy action be as likely to succeed, even though requiring more effort? Are we depriving an important client-consumer constituency of empowerment in what could be a major public issue?

Generally, advocacy aims at involvement, participation, or empowerment, and these considerations should weigh heavily if there is a fairly even choice. Obviously, there can be occasional issues where, for example, an extremely close deadline for action will preclude any mobilization of groups. Yet, if the agency's advocacy program has been following the incremental philosophy, it will find after a while that it has links to client and consumer groups that will enable it to rally them quickly and effectively.

STRATEGY

As used here, strategy refers to the selection of certain steps to reach a goal, taking into account the potentialities and constraints of the environment. Strategy consists of a series of interrelated decisions based on the study and the goals, as well as on experience, judgment, and, to some extent, guides derived from research. Generally, strategy involves consideration of the type of approach in terms of conflictual level, possible points of intervention in the target system, selection of appropriate techniques of intervention, the time and sequence framework of action, and the participation by agency and others in the action.

The first step in setting strategy is usually in the tentative determination of the conflictual level; this guides the next steps, although revisions in the level of conflict may be indicated as the planning goes through the subsequent steps.

Conflictual level. Although many conceptualizations of strategy are offered in the literature, the simplest and most practical is to see all advocacy actions on a gradient running from minimum to maximum conflict between the advocate group and the target system. Some intervention techniques are related primarily to a low conflict level, others to a moderate or high level; other techniques are neutral in relation to conflict.

As studies have shown, social workers and social work organizations favor low and moderate conflictual levels in advocacy. This is probably due to the fact that advocacy is institutionalized in the sense that agencies are established and work within a framework of other agencies and services. Some advocacy - by family agencies, for example - is seen as ongoing and generalized and directed partly toward incremental, long-term effects. Alliances with other groups, outside this system, who favor more highly conflictual strategies, may pose problems.

Within a low to moderate level of conflict, there are important variations. The level of conflict involves the inherent visibility of the advocacy action and the publicizing of it. A march on city hall is per se publicly visible. A meeting with officials may or may not have visibility. The publicizing of an action is a strategic decision; most intervention techniques can be publicized, though some are more newsworthy than others.

As a guiding principle, the decision to have a very low conflictual level will mean choosing intervention techniques that in themselves are not visible or are neutral and can be controlled. The conflictual level tends to rise with the public notice of the advocacy action. Choice of a very low conflictual level initially, however, does not preclude an escalation of level, and some intervention techniques lend themselves to this escalation. A client group and advocate can have an informal meeting with officials of the target organization, with no publicity; but if this fails to gain results, a next step could well be a public meeting or other event in which the client group testifies to the effects of the problem.

The study should yield information essential in setting the conflictual level. Information on the target organization or system can indicate points of vulnerability, usual responses to requests or demands for change, general stance in regard to change. The study also should describe any prior efforts regarding the target problem. If the target organization has not previously been approached, it is often advisable to start with a very low conflictual level, or a modified level if the target organization has been shown to be adamant in rejecting changes in relation to other problems. If history shows earlier unsuccessful efforts with the problem being studied, the strategy might well call for starting at a higher conflictual level.

Intervention points. The study should indicate
the target organization decision makers in relation to the problem. Often this has to be in-
vestigated more than once. For example, officially a city commissioner may be the apparent
decision maker, but, in practice, the problem
may be resolvable at a much lower level, through
a case conference or a meeting with a middle-
management person. Or one may have to approach
one intervention point after another, when the
decision maker cannot be located from the outside.

The study should also provide information
about those on whom persons at the decision-
making level rely for support, in case counter-
actions are necessary.

Time framework and sequence of actions. Some
advocacy actions are bound to a time framework:
external deadlines such as budget hearings or
decisions, change of officials, expiration or
starting dates of laws or regulations, for example. Or the time framework may be conditioned
by the immediacy of the problem. Other advocacy
actions will not have such external boundaries,
but the plan may call for a certain pace in order to maintain momentum, adherence of support
groups, and timely publicity.

A sequence of actions, as previously discussed, may raise the conflictual level, or be a
progression at the same level but directed at
other intervention points within the target system. However, the sequence should also have a
termination point. If the planned actions do
not obtain results, the entire advocacy action
should be shelved or returned for study and complete reformulation. This, in effect, means deciding on a final conflictual level.

Participation. Chapter 2 described the various
types of manpower available for advocacy and the
process of involving them in an action. Here
the focus is on several strategic considerations
in the planning.

"Clients" refers to those who are actually
agency clients. When they are the ones who
brought the social problem to the agency's attention, the agency should generally take the
position that the clients have the problem and
the agency is there to help them tackle it.
This avoids a paternalistic posture in which the
agency takes on the problem for the clients,
leaving them outside the action· the agency may
solve the problem but at the cost of increasing
the alienation and helplessness of the clients.

"Potential clients" refers to those who have
the same problem as agency clients, and are or
may become consumers of the services in question.

"Citizens groups" are those formed by interested people who do not necessarily experience
the problem at issue.

As more consumer and citizen groups are involved in an advocacy action, the visibility of
the action increases. It becomes more known
publicly, and the conflictual level accordingly
tends to rise. The target organization or system perceives increasing public opposition and
may in turn become more resistant to change.
The planned conflictual level should therefore
accord with the scope of involvement of other
groups.

Also, as more outside groups become involved,
the complexities of working together increase.
Conflicts may develop regarding interests, leadership, and public relations. There may be de-

lays in arriving at decisions. Disagreements
may arise over the conflictual level to be
pressed. Such disagreements mean that more time
must be allowed for the process of uniting the
groups sufficiently to work together effectively.

Sometimes, because of potential conflicts
among groups, it may be decided not to bring all
into a formal coalition or other unified arrangement, but to have an informal liaison among
them in which all are directing their efforts in
various ways toward the same problem.

In the community, interest groups usually
divide into likely or unlikely allies. Likely
allies can readily be identified, as they are
already known for their positions on related
issues. Unlikely allies are those who in
certain respects may be opponents but in another
context may be potential allies. For example,
in an action for low-income housing, an agency
identified veterans' organizations as potential
allies, in that as organizations they were interested in the plight of young veterans who
could not find housing within their income
range. Local merchants also were seen as potential allies, in that many had businesses dependent on young families for income. The veterans
and merchants, however, if appealed to in their
roles as local homeowners, were strongly opposed
to low-income housing.

In contrast to the situations in which the
agency plans to involve existing groups, other
situations call for developing support groups
out of a large body of unaffiliated consumers or
citizens. For example, the agency may find that
the only organized body in the community to look
to in an action regarding a problem affecting
senior citizens is a group of middle-class retired businessmen. This group, though not hos-

tile to the issue, may not have enough commitment and understanding because they are least
affected by the problem. To relate strategy to
goals, therefore, the agency may set about developing a group more directly related to the
problem. This decision, however, affects the
planning, since much effort must first go into
locating and helping a new group to form. This
may well result in a much slower resolution of
the problem goal but a much more effective approach to the goals of participation and education.

Research has shown that it is usually unwise
to expend effort to draw in opposition groups;
much less effort is required to form a group
from among potential supporters.[1]

Selection of intervention techniques. A wide
variety of intervention techniques are described
in the next chapter. Our concern here is on
what bases should certain techniques be selected
for use.

The strategic considerations already discussed are among the main factors - conflictual level, intervention points, time framework, sequence, and participation. Other factors influ-
encing selection include:

Appropriateness. Techniques must be suited to
the nature of the issue. Some issues are already polarized at a high conflictual level;
others have a low level, with no known opponents. For example, in a given community there
does not appear to be public opposition to providing services to battered women. Educational
techniques would be useful to increase general
demand for services; confrontational techniques
would have no point.

Progression. Although the progression of actions often cannot be precisely foreseen, a plan
for strategy selects initial techniques that can
lead to next steps. Progressions may be made up
of techniques scaled to different numbers and
types of people. A plan might call first for
mailings to lists of people; a next step might
involve ads in local papers, reaching more people in a general way. Another progression might
reach various groups of people, using different
techniques for each group. Another could involve a series of groups, each of different composition, calling upon an official.

Relation of intervention technique to resources
available. This is a practical consideration -
can the agency bring together enough human resources to carry out a given intervention? For
example, a large public meeting might seem like
the best method to use, but if resources include
only a small client group and a part-time agency
staff person, it is questionable whether they
could manage it. The same consideration applies
to expertise. Is the advocacy group equipped
for a particular action? Interventions would
have to be limited unless the planning is able
to increase resources by broadening the participation.

A final consideration is how the advocacy
participants feel about possible intervention
techniques. Some may seem to fit well, others
not. Some groups may wish to stay with only
those they are used to. If participants join in
the planning of strategy, considering what most
needs to be done before settling upon specific
techniques, they will more likely be able to reconcile their preferences with the realities of
the situation.

7

METHOD: INTERVENTION

The techniques of intervention are the essence of advocacy, the specific ways of action by which an advocacy plan may reach its goal.

Despite their importance, little has been written about them. "How-to" manuals deal with the mechanics - how to organize a march, for example - with scant guidance about selecting techniques appropriate to advocacy plans. Most of the literature about advocacy is concerned only with the study and planning stages. There is a sizable body of research, but little that relates to developing strategy. Thus advocacy planners have been left on their own, in considerable measure, when they have sought answers to two significant questions:

Which techniques are most effective in relation to a certain advocacy objective? What elements need to be considered in deciding on techniques?

Intervention techniques fit into categories that are determined by the kinds of activities they represent. The range is wide, from press releases to civil disobedience. In addition, they can be rated - low, moderate, or high - on three characteristics: conflictual level, visibility, and publicity appeal.

Such ratings, of course, are only rough estimates, and vary to some extent acccording to how
the technique is used and what the stance is on an
issue. The purpose of the ratings is to call attention to the strategic considerations involved in
the selection of techniques. This provides a rough
guide to using techniques consistent with overall
strategy.

An analysis of 110 advocacy cases described in
the Family Advocacy Reporter[1] indicates that agencies tend to use low to moderate techniques, with
occasional exceptions, enabling them to be active
advocates and at the same time to retain control
over their image in the community. If strategy is
well planned, the agency is not in danger of suffering from a runaway advocacy action - which is a
common fear of those not involved in advocacy.

But the analysis also reveals that use of the
various techniques can be expanded. Involvement of
client and consumer groups, for example, is under-
used. In those advocacy cases in which client
groups were used, the conflictual level of techniques was somewhat higher. However, as Rothman
has pointed out, target organizations were found in
studies to be tolerant of higher conflictual levels
that were employed, without adverse consequences.[2]

In considering the categories of intervention
techniques, this chapter begins with advocacy
through the shaping of public opinion.

MASS MEDIA
Press, radio, and televison reach a broad public, but the advocate has only limited influence on
how they handle issues. They often present opposing points of view, which may or may not be desirable from a strategic perspective, especially if
the opposing point of view is emphasized or favorably presented. These media also are governed by

the newsworthy or human interest aspects of issues, as well as by the composition of their audience. Use of the mass media should, therefore, be carefully thought out.

Although mass media tend to both high visibility and high conflictual levels, the interest span for a given issue is usually very short. The brief burst of concentrated attention risks raising expectations of advocacy participants and the community, but may bring a solution of the problem no nearer. Thus the effect of media exposure on the target organization is unpredictable. No systematic study has been made, but it would appear that the media are particularly effective with issues involving abuses and malfunctions of organizations or systems. On polarized issues involving broader changes, media exposure may have the effect of bringing out more opposition or of solidifying the determination of the opposition.

The Press

Local community newspapers, in contrast to the metropolitan press, can be reached through press releases and submitted stories. Such papers tend not to get into controversy directly; they prefer stories oriented to local people and groups, primarily those involved in moderate community betterment efforts. The editors are often accessible, and the advocate, knowing the policies of the papers, can discuss possible coverage with them. Local papers are often read thoroughly by the people in their community and offer a good forum for an issue in whatever form the paper may be willing to use. Some papers accept feature stories, or material from which they can prepare feature stories, usually with a human interest focus. Such papers include shopper news journals, college and high school newspapers, ethnic papers, employee publications, and organizational newsletters.

The metropolitan press makes only sparing use of press releases, especially from small or unknown sources. Often a better way to obtain exposure is to hold a press conference, involving one or more persons who are newsworthy - a legislator, city official, or prominent person - as well as a client group or consumer group. This is no guarantee, however, that reporters will attend - even though advance arrangements have been made - or that much coverage will result. These drawbacks are outweighed by the attention that a good news story obtains. Contacts with the newspapers should be developed and maintained through followups, board contacts, and similar methods, so that there will be a certain readiness for the newspaper to respond when asked.

In strategy planning, it is best not to count on newspaper coverage as the vital or determining technique, since the advocate is not in control.

Television
Much of what applies to the press applies also to television. Local stations vary in their coverage of the kind of issues that human service agencies are involved in; the most frequent type of coverage is via brief news spots and in talk shows. Newscasts provide only the briefest coverage; what seemed to be full coverage during the shooting of an activity is collapsed into a minute or two in the telecast. Television coverage is perhaps most valuable in bringing the issue to the attention of many people who did not know it existed. The advocate agency should therefore follow up on television coverage with widespread publicizing of the issue to capitalize on the initial exposure. Some coverage may be obtained through educational and cable television.

Occasionally, television stations will be interested in a story on an agency program of special human interest, offering good publicity if the agency can tie in an advocacy issue. For example, a story on an agency's special services for pregnant teenagers might bring in the issue of the school system's exclusion of such girls.

Radio

Because of the limited detailed news coverage provided by radio stations, it is wise to favor an ongoing use of radio to keep an issue in the public ear, as part of a much broader publicity plan. Through stories in local papers, mailings, and fliers, an agency may publicize a radio broadcast favorable to its interests. For example, a local radio station often offered agencies a half-hour program in which to make a presentation; the half-hour, however, was on Sunday at 8 a.m., one of the least likely times to find much of an audience. However, in a wide mailing, the agency publicized the importance of the program, the speaker, and the major points. The mere fact of the broadcast occurring impresses people with its importance and and also helps sensitize them to further exposure to the issue.

Other Mass Media

Other forms of the printed word are usually less useful to an agency. Books, magazine articles, and journals only occasionally offer an advocacy opportunity. For example, something the agency is doing may be incorporated into a magazine article and can then be republicized locally through press releases or reprints. Again, this tends to place the stamp of importance on the issue, a major aim in an advocacy action.

Although it is difficult to plan for it, agency personnel may be called upon by writers for material for articles. If the agency is sufficiently alert to the opportunity and can tie an advocacy issue into the material beforehand, it may be able to obtain this type of publicity.

AUDIOVISUAL AND OTHER MATERIALS

These materials are primarily developed and distributed by the agency or by associated groups in an advocacy action. The advocacy participants control the use of such materials; they can incorporate them into the strategy, both as to content and timing. The offsetting factors are the costs involved, the problems of distribution, and the effectiveness of the coverage.

Cost of materials ranges from the low expense incurred for a mimeographed flier to an extremely high figure for a film. The use of high-cost materials is warranted only if there will be fairly prolonged usage and the means for ongoing distribution.

The problems of distribution should be planned for; a good deal of manpower is usually needed to handle mailings and telephone calling campaigns. Mailings and telephoning require the effort of compiling and correlating lists and keeping them up to date.

The design and presentation of material must be effective. Many pieces are ineffective because they lack eyecatching appeal or are confused in design, poorly written, or not geared to the intended audience. An expert should be available as a consultant if the advocate plans much use of such materials.

Fliers. Fliers are widely used in advocacy actions. They are inexpensive, quickly produced, and can be distributed by hand or as self-mailers. They are often used in conjunction with other activities, as handouts at meetings, on the street, or at certain locations; they can be distributed door-to-door. Fliers can be prepared to reflect the chosen conflictual level, from very low-conflictual-level educational,

informative pieces to high-level conflictual
material drawing sharp issues. However, fliers
often have only limited impact. Those distributed on the street are largely disregarded,
those mailed or distributed door-to-door tend to
become lost among the profusion of advertisements. Therefore, fliers may be regarded as
most effective when they are used as reinforce-
ments to other activities.

Posters. Posters obviously have a longer life
than fliers, but can offer only a limited amount
of information - usually either about an important meeting or to convey a simple concise message or slogan. Printed posters are relatively
expensive; handmade posters can be produced
cheaply. They can be displayed in a variety of
places and may well catch the attention of many
people simply by being there day after day.
However, posters, like fliers, are primarily a
technique to develop awareness, support, and
participation, rather than having a direct effect on the target organization.

Letters to community people. Letters to community people to give them information and gain
their support and participation permit a different approach than a flier. They gain effectiveness if followed by a phone call or a personal
visit.

Because of the amount of time and the number of
workers needed, the letter technique is focused
on a neighborhood or small community. Letters
usually have a specific purpose: to notify
recipients of a meeting, to invite participation, to ask their presence at a demonstration.
Preparation of letters soliciting funds should
have the benefit of a direct mail or public relations expert; some approaches are more effec-

tive than others, even though the rate of return
is rather low at best.

Bulletins and newsletters. These are good ways
to keep a constituency informed when a lengthy
advocacy action is planned. They are usually
sent to known supporters of the action, and the
mailing list is expanded primarily through new
names submitted by those already involved. Bulletins are typically focused on one point and
issued irregularly as the occasion arises; newsletters usually are sent out on a regular basis,
and cover several topics related to the issue.
Information given in such publications is public, of course, and may be conveyed to the opposition; the publications may at times be used
partly for this purpose, especially to convey
information that would not be used directly with
the target organization. For example, the advocate may wish the target organization to realize
that the advocacy action has considerable support, without conveying this directly as a
threat; a piece in a newsletter describing the
support can make the point indirectly. The adherence of influencial people may also be publicized in this way.

    Newsletters require sufficient staffing to
ensure timely production and distribution; a
newsletter that starts out regularly and then
appears only sporadically tends to convey the
message that the advocacy movement is faltering,
and supporters may lose confidence in it.

Advertisements. Advertisements in local or city
newspapers are relatively expensive and are
mainly used only at critical points and for
large-scale major issues. Ads are used primarily in two ways. One is a position statement
attested to by a number of well-known people in
the community, whose names are listed. This may

be done simply to gain further support in the community, or to bring a controversial issue into the open and raise the conflictual level. Ads may at times have secondary value; reprints can be used as mailers or fliers. Also, the attention of the mass media may be drawn to the issue, with further publicity resulting. However, obtaining the public suport of well-known people can be a time-consuming and difficult task. Usually it requires an initial core of influential people who then approach others individually, and the position statement must be drawn up in a way that it will be widely acceptable to others.

The second main way in which ads are used by a group or organization is to make its own statement of purpose. Ads can also rebut rumors or printed statements from the opposition, or to announce publicly the existence of an organized group taking a stand on a certain issue. As strategy, such ads assume that the public forum is of major importance in the action, and this assumption should not be accepted lightly. Such ads often are not answered by the oppositon, which may mean either that the public forum aspect is not important or that the ad is taken as an effort to counteract group weakness. Ads may result in drawing out opposition and polarizing the issue publicly.

Exhibits. Exhibits usually rely upon photographs or similar visual materials and hence are suitable for issues in which illustrations can convey the main message. Any accompanying text should be subsidiary; otherwise, the photographs may appear weak and unconvincing. Thus, poor housing conditions lend themselves to this type of exhibit, but delays in receiving welfare checks do not. Exhibits pose problems; the illustrations must be of high quality and well mounted, and there must be suitable places for display. Hence exhibits need the help of experts. In addition to their own merits, exhibits provide the occasion for publicity in the form of an official opening of an advocacy effort. Photographs from exhibits can also be used in fliers or posters, as well as forming part of a documentation used directly with a target organization or with decision makers.

Drama. Plays can be used effectively to develop public awareness of issues and encourage support and participation. For example, Plays for Living, from Family Service Association of America, are used to highlight a general problem; ensuing discussion relates it to the local community. The plays can be particularly effective in reaching audiences that would not respond to direct appeals or information, but are drawn in by the nature of the play.

Another type of drama, the "street drama," was used fairly widely some years ago. Impromptu plays were given on a street corner, or in buildings, to attract attention and dramatize an issue. For example, a woman and child go into a supermarket, where the child starts crying and screaming for grapes. When enough attention has been aroused, the "mother" explains to the child about the boycott of grapes now in progress. Such plays confer immediacy on an issue that otherwise may seem remote or abstract.

Tapes. Audiotapes, relatively inexpensive to produce, have limited use; getting audiences to listen to tapes is difficult, even in conjuntion with other materials. A principal use is in connection with exhibits, where tapes can convey information while people are looking at photographs or other materials.

Videotapes are more useful, though requiring expensive equipment to produce. It is important also to have professional consultation in the preparation and editing, as poorly made tapes may be ineffective. For example, wordy video-tapes primarily focused on speakers delivering a message usually do not attract much attention. Videotapes of people in their own settings de-scribing the effects of a problem in their own lives are much more dramatic and appealing.

Films and filmstrips. Because of the high cost of production and the equipment and expertise required, films and filmstrips generally are in-appropriate for agencies to make. However, many commercially produced films and filmstrips on a wide variety of topics are available; these can be used in the say way as Plays for Living. They provide an unusually good way to reach cer-tain groups, such as PTAs.

MEETINGS

Conferences, workshops, teach-ins. This type of meeting generally has an educational emphasis, with a low conflictual level. The immediate audience is often composed of workers and volun-teers already interested in the issue because of activity in related areas. Thus conferences and workshops are often used to foster commitment, to lead up to the formation of a support group, or to channel people into established groups. Some conferences can command media attention, especially by means of a well-known speaker or the presentation of newsworthy material. The visibility of conferences and workshops is rela-tively low, as they are not in an open setting. A march, in contrast, is highly visible.

Information meetings. Coffee klatches, cocktail parties, small gatherings in a neighborhood home, and similar meetings are usually aimed at

108

increasing support and participation, and at
education. The typical format is that of one or
more informal speakers from the advocate group,
followed by questions and discussion. This type
of meeting is geared primarily to neighborhood
or small-community residents; it is an important
and often very effective means of developing
grass roots involvement. As with other methods
of fostering participation, however, such meetings must provide a framework into which re-
cruits can be fitted so that their interest is
not lost through long delays in getting started.

Speakers. The advocacy group can send speakers
to the meetings of other organizations and
groups. Depending on the circumstances, this
form of activity can be aimed at educating or
involving people, or it can be direct advocacy
effort in which the conflictual level may be
fairly high. The visibility and publicity value
of this activity depends on the sponsoring organization; helpful publicity often results. A
speakers' bureau arrangement can undergird an
extensive campaign to approach many similar
groups. For example, speakers can go to all
senior citizen groups on an issue concerning the
elderly.

Rallies, protest meetings. These meetings
generate high visibility, high publicity, and a
moderate-to-high conflictual level. They serve
a dual purpose: as an intervention tool in
themselves, through publicity and visibility,
and to enhance education, morale, and recruitment. They require much preparatory work and a
substantial number of supporters who will bring
others to the meeting. A rally or protest meeting may also also be linked directly with a
march, a delegation to officials, or a demonstration at a building. Such meetings usually
represent an escalation of advocacy strategy,

rather than an initial move. A period of concentrated followup - newsletter, bulletins, ongoing activities - avoids the danger of rapid
attrition of interest and support after a massive effort.

FORMED GROUPS

This refers to groups recruited and formed, or
called together, by the advocate and advocacy associates. Although such groups usually are a means
toward an advocacy end, sometimes the mere fact
that the activity becomes known acts as an intervention tool. A target organization, becoming
aware of organizing activity, may decide to negotiate or offer acceptable solutions rather than face
organized public opposition. The opposite can also
occur, however, with the public polarization leading the organization to harden its position. Some
types of groups have more inherent visibility than
do others; for example, a small group of clients or
consumers has low visibility, whereas a coalition
of many agencies rapidly becomes known and has high
visibility.

Client group. This refers to people known to
the agency who share a common problem as individuals or groups. A client advocacy group may
arise out of a prior or concurrent group, such
as a family life education group that develops
an advocacy issue it wants to pursue. The formation of a group from a core of individual
clients (case to cause) may be difficult; the
agency may have contact with only a few such
clients, though it is obvious that many more
people have or potentially have the same problem. Reaching enough of these others to constitute a group can require extensive effort. The
task can be relatively easy if the issue is
neighborhood centered, but if the clients and
potential clients are widely scattered, the issue will have to be publicized. An agency may

also take up a public issue, whether local, statewide, or national in nature; the study phase would then have to determine what type or types of groups could be involved.

As already discussed, the participation goal is extremely important, both for the participants and for the resolution of the issue; client (or consumer) groups foster empowerment of the people involved, so that the effort expended in the development of such groups should be viewed not merely as a step toward the resolution of a problem but also as working toward the participation goal.

Consumer group. This term refers to people who have a common problem, or potentially have the problem, but are not agency clients. Such a group may come into being, for example, when the agency takes up a public issue in which some people have a complaint against an organization or system. The development of a consumer group poses some of the same problems as that of a client group. In addition, the lack of any direct connection to the agency may make it more difficult in some instances to interpret the role of the agency to potential participants. Once formed, consumer groups can function in the same ways as a client group.

Citizen group. This kind of group consists of interested people in the community who do not have the problem but want to become involved out of conviction. While such groups can be highly effective, there is often a potential danger that their interests may not sufficiently coincide with those of a client or consumer group and their support may weaken. In some situations, formation of a group of such people may be unadvisable; it would be preferable to recruit individual persons to work in the advocacy

effort. A group of concerned citizens who are
influential may, of course, be effective in some
situations, not as an ongoing group, but rather
as a group for the purpose of endorsing a
position, as in a newspaper advertisement.

Advisory group. These are groups for ongoing
activity rather than for a single advocacy action. The advisory group or committee may or
may not be active; in either case it lends credibility to activities. Such groups provide a
role for influential people in an action largely
made up of client or consumer groups, without
the possible danger of assuming leadership or,
in effect, taking the action away from the other
groups.

Task force, ad hoc group. These groups work on
specific aspects of a problem and are composed
of people who may not work together under other
circumstances. A task force usually implies an
end product, completion of a job, often within a
time framework. It is often used to carry out a
study with recommendations or plans; the study
then forms a platform for an advocacy action. A
task force can be made up of people from various
groups and organizations. An ad hoc group, as
its name implies, is primarily a temporary committee set up within an organization but, if the
organization is a council of agencies, the committee will be made up of representatives from
diverse groups. In planning, a task force or ad
hoc committee would usually do its work near the
beginning of an advocacy action and be related
to further study, planning, and education
goals. The conflictual and public visibility
levels are usually low; they may have moderate
publicity value.

Interagency committee. This type of committee
is somewhat similar to an ad hoc committee in

that it usually is temporary and focused on a
specific issue. It may include representatives
of the target organization or system, but not
client or consumer participation since agencies,
rather than other groups, participate. Some interagency committees are informal in that agencies are not represented officially, and because
they are designed for educational purposes and
to influence staff of other agencies. The conflictual level is low, as are visibility and
publicity.

Coalition. This is an alliance of groups and
organizations, with a focus on one general issue
or concern. A coalition may deal with various
problems within the general concern - for example, a coalition on welfare reform would take up
a wide variety of facets of welfare reform as
well as maintaining a pressure for reform per
se. Coalitions can be informal, or formalized
with their own structure and even staff.

An informal coalition enables several groups
to work together toward common objectives, but
without any organization or public presentation
of an alliance as such. The purpose is usually
to achieve some coordination of strategy and action, pooling the strengths of each group. Formal coalitions may develop out of such informal
alliances.

Formal coalitions are increasingly being used
to mobilize forces for change. Research literature offers little on the process and practical
aspects of coalition building. One helpful publication, a brochure entitled A Practical Guide
to Coalition Building, outlines briefly the major premises of coalition building, leadership,
and maintenance.[3] Several of the premises are:

  - coalitions can be temporary or permanent

- individual groups retain identity and autonomy
- each group should see the coalition as capable of achieving what a group cannot do on its own
- internal group conflict is inevitable and should be seen as part of the process of coalition building

A formal coalition can carry significant weight in advocacy, but much effort is required to build and maintain a coalition. Sometimes one or more member groups assign staff time to the coalition to help it function. Its conflictual level can vary from low to high. Visibility is usually low to moderate; publicity value is often moderate to high. A coalition has the marked advantage that no one member group assumes much risk and is unlikely to be singled out for reprisals.

An example of a coalition would be a coalition for day care, made up of day care agencies and other health and welfare agencies concerned with the development of day care - citizens' groups and parents' groups, for example. Public as well as voluntary organizations may belong. The coalition is often directed against a system rather than one target organization. A coalition for day care is different from a day care council, made up only of day care agencies and concerned with day care operation and related issues. A coalition also differs from a council of social agencies both in the diversity of its membership and in its more specific focus.

STUDY/ACTION

Studies and surveys contribute to the study phase of advocacy, but should also be regarded as intervention techniques in themselves. They offer many opportunities to draw in participants, and to increase their understanding and commitment.

Study. A study primarily gathers available data on the problem. It often culminates in a report that pulls together the information in a usable form, together with conclusions and recommendations. A full study may embody the results of other data-collecting methods, described below. A study group can, with much effort, operate without guidance, but usually a person with knowledge and experience gives some direction as to sources of information, the kinds of information needed, and some help in ways of evaluating information. This guidance may be provided by the family advocate or an agency staff member assigned to work with a group.

The conflictual level of a study is obviously low, as is its visibility; however, some studies, when completed, may provide a good basis for publicity and the launching of an advocacy action.

Survey. This is used for the development of firsthand or direct information, usually through methods such as interviewing and sampling opinions. A survey of family violence, conducted in one community through telephone calls to a substantial number of randomly selected families, produced information not previously available in the community. A survey can, of course, be encompassed within a larger study. Surveys have a low conflictual level, but moderate to high visibility, and often have considerable publicity value.

Surveys may arouse opposition, however, since many communities have been oversurveyed. This has happened especially in low income or minority areas, without any action resulting. The

kinds of questions asked, or not asked, often
seem biased against the group being surveyed.
This reinforces the point that client and community groups should be involved in advocacy
planning and action so that the entire process
ties in with the community or group.

Field visits. These may be regarded as similar
to surveys. They are made to observe conditions
in an institution, or facility, or neighborhood. In addition to generating a particular
type of material, field visits are an excellent
means of educating and drawing in potential participants. As with surveys, the visibility is
moderate to high; the conflictual level also
tends to be moderate to high, depending on the
object of the visits. For example, field visits
to nursing homes can reveal a conflictual intention on the part of the advocacy effort. Field
visits to observe deteriorated housing, however,
may not have any conflictual effect on the city
government. In some situations, publicity value
may be high, for example, when a reporter accom-
panies participants on a field visit.

Photographic study. This activity, which includes videotaping, often is coupled with field
visits to procure visual documentation for use
later. Many advocacy situations, however, cannot be documented with photographs, and any photographs obtained would serve primarily as illustrations for use in exhibits or printed materials.

Monitor or watchdog activity. Such activity is
used in two ways - one, to carry out observation
over a period in order to pinpoint problems; and
two, to observe whether changes made by a target
organization are maintained after they are in-
stituted. For instance, a group may monitor
court proceedings to isolate processes that seem

to work against people. When changes have been made in the court, the group may continue monitoring from time to time to ensure that relapses have not occurred.

Monitoring is another activity that provides opportunities to involve participants more deeply. If done openly, monitoring may have a high conflictual level and be quite visible. It is unlikely to have much publicity value. However, monitoring can in some situations be carried out without revealing the purpose, which then reduces the conflictual and visibility levels.

Demonstration projects. These activities involve study and one kind of action (usually service). Demonstration projects are in one sense advocacy oriented or at least change oriented, in that they seek to model better ways of doing things. This change orientation can be made more advocacy oriented if this purpose is incorporated in the design and if the project's functioning and results are used in advocacy. For example, an agency may sponsor a two-year project providing a combination of services to teen-age mothers in a school, following a study of the problem of the school's excluding such girls. The project can be seen as an advocacy technique if the agency then tries to have the entire school system carry out the new program in all schools.

There is considerable literature on this type of intervention. The best overview can be obtained from "Promoting Innovation and Change in Organizations and Committees,"[4] Research is reviewed, followed by case examples started and studied for this purpose. A number of generalizations or principles derived from research are described. A more detailed description can be found in Planning and Organizing for Social

Change[5] which is based primarily on Rogers's
Diffusion of Innovation.

DIRECT CONTACT WITH DECISION MAKERS
This section encompasses those techniques that
bring an advocacy group into direct contact with a
target organization on the level of discussing
changes or working on the changes.

Case conference. Such a conference is held between the advocate agency or group and the target organization on individual cases or typical
cases in an effort to change current waysof
handling them. The technique relies primarily
on persuasion and appeal to professional ethics
or humane considerations. While the actual decision maker may not be at such conferences, by
implication his or her permission has been
granted to hold the conference, and the actual
decision may be made by middle management - a
case supervisor or department head. A case conference may bring about the desired results, or
it may reveal the necessity for advocacy action
or for increasing the pressure for change by
other means. The conflictual level of a case
conference is inherently low (although it may
rise as inability to reach agreement escalates);
visibility and publicity value are obviously
very low. Thus, a case conference represents a
low-keyed approach.

Negotiation. This term refers to give-and-take
discussions with decision makers or their representatives, aimed at reaching agreement on
changes. They can occur at any point during an
action; often an initial attemp is made before
resorting to other techniques. But negotiation
also occurs as the final step, since the aim of
other techniques is to bring the target organization into negotiation on terms favorable to
the advocacy group. In some advocacy actions,

of course, face-to-face meetings do not occur;
negotiations may be be conducted by letter or
telephone. In some instances the target organization announces a change as a result of being
influenced by other techniques without direct
contact.

Negotiations may be conducted by a single
representative or by a delegation from the advocacy group. The meetings may be informal, with
open discussion and give-and-take. Formally arranged and structured meetings usually arise out
of a higher conflictual level, often with higher
visibility and publicity.

Careful preparation is requred for all negotiating, with documentation organized and sound-
ly based. It is also important to be aware of
the target organization's likely arguments and
justifications for its position. The latter information should have been developed during the
study phase or acquired later and added to the
study materials.

Administrative redress. Formalized redress is
usually limited to individual cases; typically,
the client is allowed to bring a representative
or advocate to assist. An advocacy action may
plan to bring several similar cases before the
formal administrative appeal mechanism, not only
to comply with necessary procedures, but also to
determine whether success with individual cases
will bring about a policy change in the target
organization. Because such appeal mechanisms
often drag out for long periods before a decision is rendered, advocacy action may be planned
to continue during the waiting period. It
should be noted that success with an administrative appeal does not guarantee a policy change,
as many organizations focus on singular circumstances in a given case and deny that it has

general applicability. With many governmental agencies, the decision on an appeal or fair hearing is actually made at the next higher level, and again may have little effect on local practice or policy.

Public hearings conducted by target organizations. Many public agencies are now required to hold public hearings on plans and budgets; this provides a forum for advocacy, since officials are present. Hearings may be covered by the press, giving additional strength to the action. The conflictual level can be varied by the advocate, ranging from a low level focused on information giving and persuasion, to a high conflictual level in which outright opposition is expressed. The latter is usually backed up by mustering a large supporting group to attend the hearing. Both the visibility and the publicity value can be high, especially if the advocate group can make a dramatic presentation.

Consultation and training in the target organization. This can be done, obviously, only with the sanction of the organization, indicating a tacit or explicit agreement that change is needed. While consultation and training can be seen as service rather than advocacy, if it is done as part of an advocacy plan it can be regarded as the working out of the plan, especially since it is aimed at producing changes in the target organization. As an intervention technique, it is low keyed.

PUBLIC OPPOSITION

Some intervention techniques are intended to show publicly the opposition of the advocacy group. The conflictual level thus ranges more frequently from moderate to high, as is true of the visibility level and, often, the publicity value of the technique. Some techniques are clearly much stronger expressions than others.

Petitions. This technique has much value in involving participants in an action, and also in bringing the issue to the attention of individuals through personal contact and discussion. If is often used fairly early in an advocacy action. By itself, a petition tends to have relatively little force; officials and politicians have become accustomed to receiving petitions and to discounting their significance. However, when part of an overall plan and followed up by other techniques, petitions can have effect. Planners of an advocacy action should weigh advantages and disadvantages, however, and the large-scale effort required to obtain an impressive number of signed petitions may be out of keeping with the manpower available or needed for other techniques.

Resolutions. As with petitions, the force of resolutions is often small. They put the target organization on notice that the agency or group of agencies or other groups are taking a position in opposition to the target organization. If relationships have previously been fairly cooperative or neutral, the target organization may sometimes take this as the occasion to accept negotiations. Resolutions directed to a state government or the federal government, however, are in effect seen much as petitions, signed in this case by organizations rather than individuals. The conflictual level may vary; visibility is generally low, as is the publicity value.

Expert testimony. Testimony is often given by a staff member of an agency before a committee of a legislative body, and as such is an activity that belongs in this book's discussion of political and legislative techniques. Expert testimony may also be given at organized hearings or before local governmental bodies. Testifying provides a valuable opportunity for placing an issue before the public, from a position of some strength. The role of expert usually calls for a low to moderate conflictual level, however, in the content of the testimony. A transcript of the testimony, with accompanying charts and pictures, also can provide the basis for mailings and other publicizing of the information.

Organized hearings. The agency or advocate can organize its own hearing at which clients, consumers, and others may testify. Although it is obviously one-sided, it can have a very dramatic effect. Such hearings can have moderate to high conflictual level, and do have and are meant to have high visibility and publicity.

Letter/telephone campaign: persistent demands. Letters and telephoning are directed to the target organization (or its support system), in contrast to the use of letters and others means to reach the community for education and participation. The campaign may call for letters or phone calls from certain persons to the target organization, or the members of a large group may be urged to write or call. Frequent repetition is termed "persistent demands," in which the tone of the communications becomes more demanding and forceful. An extreme version is "harassment," in which, for example, the switchboard of the target organization is tied up by a large volume of calls, or officials are called frequently at home. This tactic may not be very effective, however, as it may signal to the target organization that the advocacy group lacks real clout and is resorting to petty nuisances. It also may stiffen opposition and provoke

retaliation. Conceivably it would be more suitable in dealing with a highly resistant organization that refuses to communicate at all with
the advocacy group. The conflictual level can
range from moderate to high; public visibility
and publicity value would usually be low.

Demonstrations. This topic includes a variety
of activities, all of which are highly visible
to the public and often command much publicity.
Marches, motorcades, and parades attract attention by moving through the streets to a destina-
tion, usually the target organization. Activity
at the target organization usually includes
picketing, that is, marching back and forth
carrying signs, passing out literature, making
speeches to the public. Similar tactics include
vigils and fasts.

Large-scale demonstrations require great
planning capacity, mobilization of people, plus
many provisions for safety and order. People
often need transportation, food, and emergency
medical care. Demonstrations are most frequently mounted against legislators or state officials, though some are directed at city governments. Despite the apparent strength and determination of the participants, their impact on
legislators is uncertain unless backed by a combination of other intervention techniques.
Demonstrations have considerable value for the
participants, and can result in bonds among
them. Yet there is the danger, as with mass
meetings, that the energy and enthusiasm can
quickly dissipate unless there is followup with
the participants.

Demonstrations are usually at a high conflictual level, with high visibility and publicity
value.

Civil disobedience (potential and actual). One
of the most frequent varieties of potential
civil disobedience is the "ins" - sit-in,
teach-in, camp-in. If conducted on the premises of the target organization, they can become legal violations if the participants are
asked to leave and refuse. Often target organizations are reluctant to take such measures as
calling the police to forcibly evict the participants and then pressing charges. However,
this risk does exist, and the agency and all
participants should be aware of it. Such activities obviously rate high in conflictual level,
visibility, and publicity value.

Another form of potential civil disobedience
is the refusal to comply. This arises at times
out of the nature of the problem itself, and represents the only tactic available in time to
prevent an undesired result. In one case, for
example, a large number of agencies were noti-
fied they must submit certain data to the funding organization starting on a fixed date. The
agencies objected that disclosure of the data
would violate client rights and possibly put
clients in jeopardy of the law. They all refused to comply. The target organization did
not press for compliance in the face of this opposition, although it could not only have termi-
nated contracts but possibly have involved the
agencies in legal processes relating to laws
concerning drug users. A suitable compromise
was reached.

Refusal to comply is not civil disobedience
per se, unless the matter is ruled so by a court
interpreting the law. However, in some instances refusal to comply may be in clear violation
of law, and may be so intended by an advocacy
group as an effort to challenge the law and
press for change. Such protests often can

result in fines or jail terms, as occurred in the civil rights movement.

It would seem unlikely that human service agencies would frequently resort to civil diso- bedience as a planned intervention technique, although, as in the example above, it might be necessary occasionally. Such agencies tend to use intervention techniques that do not register the highest ranges of conflictual level, visibi- lity, and publicity; their stance is that of re- form rather than radical change. This position is consonant with the fact that human service agencies are part of the established support network in a community and must continue their range of services.

Creating internal pressure in the target organi- zation. Much has been published about changing an organization from within, ranging from alter- ing goals to modifying attitudes of personnel. Techniques to influence the organization from the outside by creating pressure are less under- stood and infrequently used. For example, it is conceivable to persuade one or more board mem- bers of the target organization to resign, mak- ing public statements. This action would presu- mably create considerable disturbance within the board and the rest of the organization. How- ever, if the situation is seen as a factional struggle within the organization, such an action is unlikely to influence the "victors." Another technique is that of creating disaffection among employees by appealing to professionals within the target organization, on the basis of profes- sional ethics, to carry out some form of action within the organization, or to influence other employees to carry out some action - a slow-down or "sick-out," for example. Its effectiveness would seem to hinge upon the prior development of sufficient feeling of solidarity of personnel

with the cause and with people outside the organization.

While this tactic may not be used often as a
technique, the case conference method may. In
one agency program, frequent case conferences
took place between agency staff and staff from
the department of social services. As the latter learned more and understood the content as a
different way of regarding clients, they in turn
brought pressure to bear upon their agency to
institute changes that were not restricted to
the subjects of the conference.

Court action. While agencies generally are not
equipped to carry a case to court, they do on
occasion work with lawyers on advocacy issues.
Lawyers will usually try to negotiate first,
bringing to bear their special expertise. Recourse to the courts, however, brings in other
factors that should be considered carefully.
Court action tends to draw sharp lines of opposition and often makes other intervention techniques useless until the court decision is rendered.

Court action has several other possible drawbacks that enter into advocacy planning. First,
court action tends toward a win-or-lose resolution, so that possibilities of compromise are
lessened. On the other hand, court action can
have the effect of bringing the opposition to
the negotiating table. The effect of a successful court outcome may not be as extensive as
hoped for. Unless a class action suit is
brought, a court ruling on one case may not lead
to a policy change by the target organization,
which may return to court several times to test
whether a general rule is involved, at the cost
of much time and stress. And court decisions
may be appealed by either side, so that a long

period may ensue before a final verdict is given. This delay can vitiate an advocacy group.

Notwithstanding these considerations, there are important situations in which the courts become the only recourse for change. In one state, for example, the legislature enacted a residency law for welfare recipients, despite massive advocacy efforts. Within a short time, an injunction was obtained suspending implementation until a court decision was reached. After appeals, the state government lost. The next year, however, a somewhat changed bill was enacted and a second court action was necessary. Although this law also was found unconstitutional, further attempts at legislation were made. Obviously, the political forces were far stronger in the legislature than the advocacy forces, and the only countervailing force was repeated legal action.

In planning, consultation with lawyers or with a legal service for low-income people is important to determine whether clients' rights are involved, and whether legal action is indicated and can be brought. If possible, the agency should involve a lawyer in its advocacy committee or as an advocacy associate available to the advocate. There are gray areas in which legal action may be possible but where other factors make recourse to it questionable. Clients or other groups have the right to be fully informed then, so that they can arrive at a decision.

ADVOCACY, POLITICS, AND GOVERNMENT

Advocacy for human services is facing new and
severe challenges in the political arena. Law
making and administration affecting those services
in the past was confined largely to one level, the
federal government. In recent years, there has
been movement into state and local levels, a movement that became an avalanche with Reaganomics,
block grants to states, and the new federalism.
Although the avalanche may melt away, its effect
will be long-standing. The movement from centrali-
zation to decentralization is one of the major directions of society in our time, according to John
Naisbitt in Megatrends: Ten New Directions Transforming Our Lives. In his view, Ronald Reagan is
not responsible for the new federalism; he is merely "riding the horse in the direction the horse is
going."[1] Because of the trend - which Naisbitt
applauds - state and local governments are becoming
involved in social services in new ways, with additional fiscal and policy-making authority and with
increased responsibility. Advocates for human service organizations need more than ever before to be
able to function effectively on the state and local
levels. It is essential that they influence the
ways in which block grants - which the states wel-
come - are used by state governments. Advocates
need to be persuasive as states act out their new
roles in defining and funding social services.
They need to provide assistance, insight, and

perspective as states strive to develop the planning and research capabilities and taxing authority required of them.

THE STATE LEGISLATURE

A specific point of reference for discussing advocacy in the political arena today is the state legislature, where laws are made that affect millions of people and hundreds of local communities. Its members are sensitive to powerful constituencies, which indicates the importance to human service organizations of building coalitions representing large numbers of voters. Advocates will provide expert advice on drafting bills. In local communities, individual agencies will represent their views to their local legislative representatives. Some of the intervention techniques described in preceding chapters can be utilized.

An essential ingredient in advocacy today is clear understanding of the workings of the state legislative process. Such understanding will help advocates to determine when intervention will be most effective. The following description of the process that follows is condensed from an article in Child Welfare, written by Maureen Hassett Herman and Brendan V. Callanan:[2]

The reasons legislation fails or passes are as varied as the array of state legislators. Yet there are definite steps that can be taken at certain junctures of the legislative process that will invariably exert a significant influence on the course of legislation. A comprehension of the legislative process enables advocates to time their efforts appropriately, and not waste them on bills that have already been voted on or have languished in committee past the deadline for legislative consideration. The selection of methods in working for legislation is also important. Too often an advocate considers a flood of form letters to legislators as a primary influence. However, lobbyists consider letter-writing campaigns largely ineffectual. The lobbyists' view is usually accurate if these letters are not appropriately timed and not used in conjunction with other tactics.

Following is a description of how a bill is enacted into law (the 50 states' legislative procedures vary, but not substantially):
1) Initiation of bill
2) Introduction of bill by member
3) Referral of bill to committee
4) Committee action
   a) Hearing: open, for testimony, or closed, possibly for deliberation, amendment, and decision
   b) Common recommendations: that the bill does pass, does not pass, does pass as amended, be indefinitely postponed, be recommitted to another committee without recommendation (sometimes this is not permitted)
5) Floor debate and action
   a) Rejection or acceptance of committee amendments and recommendations
   b) Other amendments
6) Same five steps in the other house; if the bill is amended, it is returned to the other house for ratification or sent to a conference committee
7) Governors' action
   a) approve
   b) veto, bill then goes back to legislature for another vote
   c) permit bill to become law without signature.

Awareness of the steps in the legislative process allows advocates to exert pressure and provide information at the crucial time in that

process. They can influence whether a bill
passes or fails, particularly if the suggestions
that follow for each major step in statute making are implemented.

Initiation of the Bill

A problem is identified by either an individual, an agency, or an organization. An analysis should be made of existing and proposed
methods to solve it. The credibility of a witness who is unaware of prior attempts to rectify
the situation either by existing statutes or
pending legislation is destroyed. It is necessary to be able to explain why existing laws are
inadequate. For example, at a recent state committee hearing a witness was not cognizant of
the effects of a bill, passed only the year before, to provide for insulation in low income
housing, the identical purpose of the bill the
witness was advocating. One cannot operate in a
vacuum and expect success. However, recognition
of a need for legislation and understanding of
the inadequacy of the present statutes are rare-
ly enough by themselves to get a bill passed.
Legislators, as all of us, are aware of many deficiencies in existing statutes. A remedy for
these imperfections must be developed and proposed. It is precisely at this step that many
unnecessarily retreat. They usually have in
mind a specific way to achieve some objective,
but have misgivings about their ability to con-
vert their ideas into a written bill. If brief,
concise language is used, anyone can draft a
bill, although ideally a bill should be reviewed
by an attorney before introduction. Primarily,
bill drafting in this field requires a knowledge
of the practices and administrative structure of
the pertinent system. Bill drafting, therefore,
should not be a barrier to the continued involvement of advocates, although care must be taken
with the language. Many organizations have

available for assistance either an in-house counsel or a legal consultant. The traditional writing of bills in language incomprehensible not only to the average citizen but to the normal legislator has contributed to advocates' attitude that bill drafting is too difficult to undertake. Fortunately, there is a current trend toward use of clear, readily understandable language.

Meticulous attention to the wording of a bill and its composition is nevertheless important, since imprecise wording can be construed to have a totally different meaning from the original concept. Faulty wording of bills can make the legislators look incompetent in the eyes of their constituency. If their concern with "good image" is not taken into account, one can quickly lose their support of any measure.

In many states, once the bill is drafted it must be printed in bill form prior to introduction. This task is usually performed by the legislative council or a similar body in the legislature. The legislative council is usually a permanent, bipartisan, bicameral legislative research committee whose basic services include bill drafting, preparation of bills and law summaries, legal counsel for legislators, and revision of statutes. As the session proceeds, there is an increasing backlog of bills to be printed. This can result in several weeks' delay before a bill can be printed and hence introduced. Therefore, a bill should be printed before the session begins, or as early in the session as possible.

Coalitions are usually desirable when a bill is initially proposed. Legislators are more likely to consider a measure supported by several groups than by an individual. Meetings with groups concerned with the problem should be initiated long before a legislative session begins. It is imperative to have the groups' active support. If all appropriate organizations are involved in the beginning, problems will be minimized at hearings, where their support can be crucial.

The public agency that would be charged with implementation of the bill is often an essential supporter. Whether to strive for the agency's backing depends on the political situation in the state. In instances where the governor and the agency's administrator are politically opposed to the legislature, the administrator's support may be detrimental to passage. Otherwise, the approval of the public agency, even though it may not actively push the bill, can facilitate its course through the legislature.

Advocates should contact the legislative research bureau staff and committee staff and offer to provide information on questions about the bill. The legislative staff play a major role in some states in the selection of bills to be introduced and actively considered by the committee members. They frequently analyze the bills and problems presented and suggest to a legislator the ones they find appropriate. Research and analysis services for legislators were traditionally provided by a central legislative council or legislative reference bureau, but the trend is to provide specialized staff directly to the committees. The latest survey taken by the Council of State Governments found that professional assistance is provided to all standing committees in 35 states. This enables advocates to identify easily the staff directly assisting a particular committee. However, the legislative reference bureau of legislative council staff should also be informed of the availability of information, since they will probably draft the fiscal note on the bill and the summary of the bill.

The legislative staffs can play a crucial role in the legislative process because of the overwhelming number of issues legislators must deal with during a session. The legislators are not experts in all these diverse areas, so they rely on staff for assistance.

In the states that utilize an interim study committee, the staff is also a good starting point for a bill. Since many standing committees' terms have been extended to a full year, there has been a decrease in the use of the interim study committee in state legislatures. Depending on the subject matter, the interim study committees generally are searching for solutions to particular problems and are not subjected to the extreme time pressures of a regular session committee. Several states have set up interim committees to consolidate their laws regarding juveniles into a juvenile code. This basically involves transfer of all relevant sections of the state code into one chapter dealing specifically with juvenile matters. While recodifying these scattered statutes, the committee is also searching for improvements to them. The advocate who suggests possible amendments to this committee can find a receptive audience.

Once the tasks of analysis, bill drafting and printing, coalition building, and stimulation of interest of agencies and organizations, legislators and their staffs are completed, the bill is ready to be introduced.

Introduction of the Bill

It is always advantageous for the legislators who will introduce the bill to be identified by

the advocate before the session begins. The
sponsor can then file (introduce) the bill before the start of the session. Only five states
do not allow presession filing of bills. If the
sponsor does not prefile the bill, it should be
introduced early in the session. Because of the
pressure of short sessions (they vary from 20
legislative days to continuous sessions), bills
introduced late in the session may not be scheduled for consideration either in a committee or
on the floor. Also, a majority of states limit
the period when a bill can be introduced during
the session. Only six states have no stated
deadline.

The choice of an appropriate legislator to
introduce the bill is frequently a key factor in
the outcome. It is always imperative to find
the sponsor with the most clout.

The chairperson of the committee to which the
bill will be referred should be the first choice
as a sponsor unless he has a poor record for
sponsoring bills that are enacted or is swamped
with other bills. The chairperson's sponsorship
gives the bill the best chance to be heard in
committee, since he or she schedules the hearings. Also, chairpersons are frequently members
of the majority party, being selected in most
states on the basis of loyalty to the majority
coalition. Majority party membership of the
sponsor is particularly beneficial in competitive two-party states.

The members of the committee handling the
bill should be approached as additional sponsors
or alternatives to the chairperson. Multiple
sponsorship diminishes the chance of the bill's
receiving a negative vote or being held up in
the committee. A committee member unfamiliar
with the bill will not be as disposed to recom-

mend passage as one sufficiently convinced of
its merits to sponsor it.

If the public agency's support for the bill
has been obtained and it has decided to recommend it to the governor, the bill may be approved for the legislative package the governor
generally proposes each year to the legislature. An administration bill usually gets more
serious consideration than other bills.

Sponsorship in both houses, where permitted,
often helps speed the bill through the legislature. If a bill can move through the House and
Senate at the same time, there is a greater
prospect that it will be passed in the session
in which it has been introduced. Also, if a
House bill is detained in committee, the Senate
bill, once passed, can be brought over to the
House and have another opportunity. Whenever
bills are concurrently introduced, it is imperative to check that the language is identical;
differences result in delay. The two versions
may be sent to a conference committee, or each
bill may have to be considered separately again
by both houses.

Referral of Bill to Committee

Once the bill is introduced, it is referred
to a committee for action. Choice of the committee is determined by the speaker of the House
and the president of the Senate in a majority of
states, and this referral is also restricted by
rules of procedure in several states. However,
there is usually some latitude as to which committee will get the bill, since jurisdictions of
the many committees overlap. Assignment to a
committee whose decisions on bills are influential can be an important factor in the bill's
disposition. Therefore, if latitude exists in
the assignment of the bill, the advocate and

sponsor should determine which committee is the best choice, and suggest this committee to the persons charged with the referral.

The committee can disregard, defeat, accept and report out, amend and report out, or rewrite the bill. It is generally in the committee that a bill's fate is decided. The power of a committee varies from state to state. A "do pass" recommendation of a weak committee cannot be relied on solely to carry a bill through the House or Senate. A bill with a "do not pass" vote, however, even from a weak committee, faces an uphill struggle.

The advocate can have a significant effect on the bill's course at the committee stage, but this involves the detective work of determining when the hearing will be held. Notice of committee hearings is posted in most states, but sometimes not until the actual day of the hearing. There is suspicion that committees discourage persons and groups from appearing at hearings by failing to publicize the time and place of such hearings. The chief clerk of the House or Senate can provide information on the bill's place on the calendar and the committee staff or chairperson on the hearing schedules. Also, the sponsor should be able to keep the advocate posted on the bill's progress. The Council of State Governments' publication Principal Legislative Staff Offices is an excellent contact tool; it identifies the key legislative functions and gives the names, addresses, and phone numbers of the legislative staffs in each state.

To testify as a witness on a bill usually requires only appearing at the hearing, but the sponsor should be told who intends to appear and the issues each witness will address. This in-

formation enables the sponsor to coordinate efforts by several witnesses and to prepare his or
her opening statement. At committee hearings
other members of the House or Senate have first
priority to be heard, followed by high officials
of the pertinent public agencies, and private
citizens or groups.

An appearance is frequently damaging if not
properly prepared for. The provision of written
and oral testimony on the bill is important but
testimony must meet the following criteria.

1) Accuracy. Know the basis for the information presented and collect data to support the
testimony. Research should be done beforehand.
The fiscal note prepared on a bill by the legislative staff contains an estimate of the cost of
the bill, and this should be obtained and analyzed before an appearance at a committee hearing. An advocate should be prepared to answer
questions on fiscal impact. For many legislators, this is a paramount concern.

2) Balance. Realize that the bill is not an
all-encompassing solution to the problem, but
specify exactly what it does and does not pro-
pose to accomplish. The committee members are
not experts in all matters, but will be receptive to expert testimony if it is not too
slanted.

3) Thoroughness. As already stated, an analysis should also be made of the existing laws
and administrative procedures that deal with the
same concern. Basic facts on how existing statutes deal with the problem or on the lack of
relevant laws are important.

4) Brevity. A grave mistake at committee
hearings is for a witness to describe everything

in minute detail. The aim should be to answer precisely the questions that committee members raise. A brief description of the purpose of the bill, with time reserved for questions, is usually the best approach. If the bill is discussed on the floor, it is important to have educated the committee members as to the bill's merits. Their questions must be answered in the committee hearing, since the witness will not be able to speak up on the floor if questions arise; that will be the sponsor's responsibility.

5) Appropriateness. An identification of the backgrounds of the committee members can enable a witness to prepare testimony tailored to their interests. A committee largely composed of attorneys will be receptive to a witness who explains the legal ramifications of the bill. Listings of state legislators, with background information on each, are available in states through a variety of sources, including lobbying associations and the state itself.

Committees handle many diverse bills in an average day. Therefore, many legislators have not had time even to read the bill under consideration. This makes fact sheets on the major purposes of the bill helpful. The fact sheets should be circulated before as well as at the time of a hearing.

A bill passed favorably out of committee, particularly by a unanimous vote, has a good chance to survive a floor vote. State legislators frequently must rely on the committee report, due to time limitations, their own concerns, and lack of staff. The committee stage of the legislative process is one where advocates can have a strong effect on the course of a bill.

Floor Debate and Action

Once the bill is reported out of committee, it is scheduled for a floor vote. A calendar or steering committee or some similar committee of chairpersons of committees in both houses or the legislative leadership decides on the calendar of bills to be heard on the floor. At this point the sponsor or advocate can try to exert influence by contacting a member of this committee. If personal contacts fail and the session is about to end, letters from constituents of the committee members might expedite scheduling of the bill. States usually just list the bills to be heard on the floor that day.

In 12 states the committees hearing a bill must report on all bills assigned to them, but the committees in the remaining states can pigeonhole a bill by not acting on it. The earlier a bill is reported out of committee, the greater the opportunity for it to be placed on the calendar for a floor vote.

A bill will often be defeated if intense controversy develops in the floor debate. Therefore, in this situation, it is often wise for the sponsor to suggest that the bill be referred back to committee before a vote is taken. Problems arising on the floor provide clues concerning which members to contact before the next session. Personal contacts to answer the objections of the protesting members are usually more effective than written communications. A coordination of efforts with the bill's sponsor is important. An effective approach is for the sponsor to speak with the opposing members, and then have the advocates follow up with written analyses and further answers to specific questions.

Most states have daily records of legislative proceedings, but sometimes the record is limited to actions already taken, with no reports on the debates. In states where records of the debates are available, they can be consulted to determine which factors motivated the bill's defeat or referral back to committee. These journals are particularly helpful when attendance at the debate is not possible. Efforts should then be directed at those members with the strongest objections and at the issues identified for study by the committee to which the bill was reassigned. When a bill has been referred to committee or not voted on, a few states allow it to be carried over automatically to the next session. If not, the bill should be introduced early in the next session or prefiled.

Preceding Steps Repeated in Other House

A bill passed by one house is sent to the other house. (There is only one state with a unicameral legislature - Nebraska.) In the other house, the bill goes through the same process already described. The advocate must again make known the availability of information, testify at the hearing, provide written materials on the bill, and monitor the bill's course. If the bill is amended, it will be sent back to the originating house to be ratified. The bill is sent usually to a conference committee of members of both houses if the two houses fail to agree on amendments. Once agreement is reached in this committee, its report is usually accepted by both houses.

Governor's Action

After the bill has been passed by each house, it is sent to the governor, who can sign it, disregard it, or veto it. In some states, after a stipulated number of days a bill becomes law unless vetoed. If the bill is vetoed, procedures exist for an overriding vote. The political situation between the governor and the two houses greatly influences the likelihood of an overriding vote. The vote required in the House and Senate to pass a bill over a veto ranges from three-fifths of members present to three-fourths of those elected. North Carolina is the only state in which the governor does not have veto power. A bill that is signed usually becomes effective on a specified day, often 90 days after the legislature adjourns.

Implementation
Once the bill has been passed, the work of an advocate has really only begun. Those advocates who worked for the passage of legislation must continue to devote their attention to its successful implementation. If all interest dissipates upon enactment of the bill, the administrative machinery necessary to put it into action can be slow and dysfunctional. First, to speed up the administrative process, an informational bulletin for the groups affected by its provisions and a press release to the general public should be prepared by the advocate and submitted for release by the administrative agency. Also, appropriate action by the agency to carry out the bill's mandates can be encouraged by the advocate's suggestions and surveillance of agency implementation.

THE PROCESS VARIES
Since the legislative process varies from state to state, it is very important for advocates to be well informed about the detailed workings of their own legislatures. This point is made by Joan W. Lawrence, who worked as an advocate for human service agencies before becoming a member of the Ohio House of Representatives.

Ms. Lawrence does not agree that letter-writing campaigns are completely ineffectual. "Volume of mail matters," she says, "and is much better than nothing." She feels that a legislator should be involved even before a bill is initiated - if possible, at the time when a problem needing legislation is identified. In regard to drafting legislation, she says, "In Ohio, we would not expect - or even want - advocates to draft legislation. It is better if they prepare good outlines of concerns and situations. Drafting can be done better by professional legislative staff, once a legislator to carry the proposal is found."

In the critical period when a bill is scheduled for floor vote, according to Ms. Lawrence, an advocate may want to poll the legislative body in advance if there seems some likelihood that conditions are not right for passage. If the poll does indicate a problem, it may be possible to have the vote delayed until a time when passage is possible.

Janet Bernon of the Center for Human Services in Cleveland, Ohio, is also widely experienced as an advocate. Like Ms. Lawrence, she believes that letter writing is a valuable tool, but she discriminates between form letters and personal letters from constituents to individual legislators; the latter are much more effective than the former, in her opinion.

Ms. Bernon emphasizes that an attempt to have a bill enacted should begin with the advocate's finding a key supporter for it in the legislature. The step should be taken before the bill is drafted, in her judgement. At that stage, the legislator needs only to understand the intent of the proposed legislation.

She puts a high value on interpreting a bill to lawmakers in terms of its impact on people. Advocates appearing as witnesses before a committee need specific, detailed information about people to support their testimony. If the advocates prepare a description of the purpose of the bill, the description should explain the impact on people if the bill is enacted.

If a bill is approved in committee, it moves to a steering committee that will decide when it is to come before the legislative body. A bill can get bogged down in the committee; if the advocate determines to try to move it out by contacting a committee member, Ms. Bernon advises that the contact be made by someone who is one of the committee member's constituents.

Maxine Selling, family advocate of Metropolitan Family Service, in Portland, Oregon, believes in the importance of working with the legislatures' interim committees. In her state, the legislature has an Emergency Board during the interim:

"Membership on it consists of the Joint Ways and Means Committee from the regular session. Special programs requiring emergency funding or innovative model programs have a way of receiving funding from the Emergency Board. There are fewer demands on the board, "pockets" of money held in reserve for emergencies seem to be available even in revenue-short times for sound and worthy programs. So this interim period may sometimes prove more productive than a regular legislative session for getting funds for a significant program which, during the regular session, may become drowned in the mass of bills coming to a committee."

MONITORING LEGISLATIVE ACTIVITY

A very important advocacy activity regarding legislatures is keeping in touch with bills that are supported by other interests in the state and that bear on social issues. It is important to obtain information about such items as quickly as possible, to identify those that seem to have a good chance of passage, and to decide what advocacy strategy is pertinent in supporting, amending, or opposing them. Knowledge of the legislative process will be helpful in plotting strategy and carrying it out.

AFTER A BILL BECOMES LAW
An advocate's watchfulness and inquisitiveness are never more necessary than after a bill has been passed and the resulting law is being administered.

"Monitoring the rules is the most critical part of advocacy," Ms. Lawrence said. "Advocates must know how it is done." Such monitoring may show that new regulations are not consistent with the purposes that gave the initial impetus for them. "Sometimes, it is necessary to go back to the legislators to remind them of the bill's intent," according to Ms. Bernon.

The measure of an advocacy project's success is in the benefits it brings to the people it is intended to serve. Acting on this principle, an advocate works not only with the legislative branch of a state government but with the executive branch as well. The nature of this activity is described in the Government Relations Manual of the United Way of America:

At the state level you will also find state agencies carrying out a broad mandate for action in their particular area. Often staff of these agencies have tremendous responsibility and authority for how state programs are run. Therefore, it is critical to determine their role within your state and to develop a good working relationship with appropriate agency staff.... Who makes decisions relative to contracting with the private sector and what are the procedures? How is the state structured to carry out its human service planning? Does it use advisory councils or regional planning committees? How can you find out about proposed policy changes?[3]

The manual makes clear the connection between state and local governments:

Each state has its own assortment of cities, counties, townships, parishes, villages, wards, and towns. Likewise, each of these geographical areas has its own governing structure. In your area of service you may have city or town councils, boards of supervisors and a variety of other groups meeting regularly to determine policy for that political jurisdiction.

Since all of these various forms of local government have the potential to set policy affecting the nonprofit sector, you should become familiar with how they operate. What powers and authority do they have? How do they relate to state government or issues of interest to you? ...How are local policies determined for spending state and federal monies?[4]

New rules based on social legislation enacted by a law-making body can be made and enforced only to the extent necessary to put the law into effect. This principle limits the power of the governmental agency that makes and enforces the rules. Intervention in these activities is a valid role for advocacy. Raymond Albert, an assistant professor in the Law and Social Policy Program at Bryn Mawr College, has written that such advocacy involves analyzing regulations and presenting written and oral testimony at hearings. In addition:

Activities following participation in the hearings can be as narrow or as comprehensive as

circumstances warrant. Certain activities are
fundamental. For example, the social worker
will maintain communications with other affected
service providers and sympathetic agency staff
to keep abreast of developments. He or she will
monitor the relevant regulations and their subsequent hearings to spot actual or potential implementation problems. It will be important to
share relevant new information with agency staff
and to mobilize support among other service providers to encourage their stake in the outcome.
The worker will identify actual or potential
problems with regulatory enforcement to make the
agency aware of such breakdowns and to prepare a
foundation for any future legal challenge. And
he or she will stand ready to organize service-
provider pressure against a proposed or final
regulation.[5]

THE ENVIRONMENT FOR ADVOCACY

Whether working at the federal, state, or local
level, with lawmakers or administrators, advocates
occasionally operate in ambiguous circumstances.
They are fortunate, however, in being in a clearer
position than they were before the Tax Reform Act
of 1976 was passed, with explicit and liberal regulations regarding lobbying. Previously, the penal-
ty for violation was loss of tax-exempt status.
Sally Y. Orr, an advocate for The Association of
Junior Leagues, Inc., has summarized its effect,
writing that it "encouraged lobbying by allowing
every public charity (except church groups) to
elect to come under an amendment which:
    "Defines lobbying;
    "Permits lobbying without penalty up to a cer-
tain percentage of the organization's total annual expenditures;
    "Penalizes minor infractions by taxing lobbying
expenditures above that percentage;
    "Reserves the ultimate penalty - loss of tax-
exempt status - for repeated excessive lobbying."[6]

The 1976 act became law in a political climate
in Washington that changed rapidly when the Reagan
Administration came to power. Human service agency
advocates felt a chill wind in 1983 when the Office
of Management and Budget (OMB) moved to restrict
"political advocacy" by groups that receive federal
funds. Such a strong protest came from a coalition
of groups that the OMB withdrew the proposed rules,
but the concern persisted about the Reagan Administration's interest in hampering the lobbying activities by human service groups.

A rule outlawing lobbying is something that advocates worry about as a future possibility. A
here-and-now problem for them is the way in which
federal cuts in domestic programs lack a consistent
pattern and are being felt most severely by the
working poor.

The cuts were studies over two years by Princeton University's Urban and Regional Research Center. The study was of a sample of fourteen representative states. Following is an extract from a
report of the study in The New York Times:

The effect of the Federal cuts varied every-
where. Some cities actually received an increase in funds for programs like community development that were cut over all, while others
found their funds cut severely.

In many states funds were shifted from large
cities to smaller communities and rural areas in
programs in which authority to decide how the
money was to be spent was shifted from the Federal Government to the states.

There was confusion over Administration efforts to reduce the regulating burden on state
and local governments. The Administration en-

couraged those governments to reduce record-keeping and reporting to Washington, but many state officials felt they did not have clear assurance of being found in compliance with Federal law.

The director of the study, Richard P. Nathan, professor of public and international affairs at Princeton's Woodrow Wilson School, said the research confirmed a tentative conclusion last year, that the cuts hit the working poor hardest and were not so damaging as expected to local governments.[7]

CONSTANCY IN CHANGE

One element of constancy in the uncertain, changing relationship between politics and government on the one hand and nonprofit human service organizations on the other is people. New laws and regulations are being created and are being administered with varying effect; institutional powers are being shifted to new locations; political ideologies challenge values that formerly were supported. But the agent of change in all of these transactions is the human being. And for that reason, the most successful advocates will be those who are effective in working with people. The truth seems self-evident, but it deserves elaboration.

People in Government

As important as it is to master the details of legislative process or grasp the implications of regulations, it is at least equally important to develop good relationships with the men and women who live in the process and write or administer the regulations. Here are some basic guidelines:

The best kind of contact with a person in politics or government is face-to-face. Getting to someone in person is far better than a letter or a phone call.

Know as much as you can about the people essential to your advocacy...their backgrounds, commitments, interests.

Know as much as you can about what you are advocating; your contacts will respect you and may ask you for information.

Maintain good relationships with the "outs" as well as the "ins" for an obvious reason: their roles may change.

Respect the roles of politicians and legislators; avoid stereotyping them; do not be critical of them.

Be patient, but persevere in working with them.

Establish and maintain trust and credibility.

Be appreciative of the help you receive.

Take the position that you are trying to help a public official and do so as often as you can.

If you find that you have to compromise on an issue, do it gracefully, without imputing wrong to the forces that make compromise necessary.

Such informal, personal ways of relating to people can lead easily to other friendly but more purposeful contacts. Maxine Snelling provides examples from her experience:

Last fall, prior to the January opening of our biennial legislative session, the board of directors of our agency initiated a purely social reception for all legislators from districts in which board members vote. The message came through to the lawmakers that the board has

a vested interest in human service programs and
will be watching for appropriate measures affecting our agency's clients who, in turn, represent a constituency of clients throughout
Oregon. The reception also called attention to
our advocacy program.

Immediately upon the convening of our legislature, I meet individually with each legislator
on the legislative committees I expect to be
monitoring. I brief them on our client profiles
and on legislation which we intend to support.
I also inform them of the professional experiences and information we have available to assist them or the committee as a whole.

Numbers of People
When a large number of people or several major
organizations speak together on an issue, politicians listen. An effective way of organizing this
kind of strength is through the building of coalitions - bringing together groups of people who find
themselves natural allies in working on an issue.
The effectiveness of a national coalition was dem-
onstrated in the reaction to the OMB's attempt to
restrict political advocacy by groups receiving
federal funds. "Once the implications sank in,"
commented an editorial in The New York Times, "a
coalition of groups as diverse as the Girl Scouts
and the National Association of Manufacturers rose
up in fury. A humiliated OMB withdrew the rules,
at least for now."[8]

With human service legislation passing to the
hands of state legislatures, coalition-building is
likely to be a growth industry, for state coalitons
as well as national will be needed. A discussion
of coalitions as an advocacy tool appears in chapter 7. Further endorsement comes from the United
Way of America:

"Coalitions can be a real source of strength to your efforts. Through the contacts of other coalitions members, your resources are multiplied; you have more willing hands helping, and you share expertise and political allies. The more people you have involved in a coordinated manner, the greater are your chances of success."[9]

Volunteers Are Important

Advocating at the state and local level puts a severe burden on human service organizations in terms of personnel needs for other strategies in addition to coalition-building. Such strategies include "planning and coordinating services, seeking changes in administrative procedures, lobbying for changes in existing legislation or the development of new laws, educating the public about existing services and needs or ensuring that various groups, e.g., the handicapped, children, obtain their legal rights."[10]

The quotation is from an article by Sally Y. Orr. Ms. Orr believes that volunteers must be used in advocacy roles if human service agencies are to preserve essential services against the threat of cuts by state legislatures. She acknowledges that social workers will need flexibility to overcome some of the difficulties of working with volunteers. One of these is the fear engendered among professionals that, in a period of budget cutbacks, volunteers will be used to replace professionals. Her response is that the development of advocacy programs often provides new professional opportunities for social workers, especially those trained in planning, policy analysis, and organization.

METHOD: OTHER ASPECTS OF ACTION

The implementation of plans is the advocacy action. In the process of advocacy, however, study, planning, and action may go on concurrently, especially at the early stages of the effort. As the advocacy action continues, the study phase decreases or ends, and planning continues in the form of revisions and additions to the initial plan. The overall plan may call for a public meeting; the detailed planning for the meeting is likely to be very time consuming but cannot be done at the point of the initial plan.

Much of the literature relating to the action phase is to be found in scattered publications of the "how to" type - how to write a press release, how to organize a public meeting, how to hold a press conference. These can be helpful if the advocacy group lacks people with experience in the various skills needed.

Three other aspects of the action phase are important: review, revision, and troubleshooting.

REVIEW
Some person or small group should be in a position to know enough of the entire action to be able to review what has taken place, relate it to what is still planned, and evaluate whether changes need to be made. Review would include such questions

as: Has the advocacy thrust slowed down, and if so, why? Are motivation and interest of participants lagging? Have unexpected barriers arisen? Are time plans being met? Have intervention techniques had the expected results? Do the elements of strategy as planned still hold good? Is more information needed? What troubles have arisen, and what do they mean for the further implementation of the plan?

REVISION

Based on the review of the action, changes and additions may be called for. To make these revisions, advocates should in effect return to the planning phase, considering any changes in light of the elements of strategy and of the available intervention techniques. Reference should be made to the goals established, either to determine if changes fit in or to rethink goals.

Quick responses and shifts in plan are often called for by external events. Yet even quick responses should be subjected to the same process of rethinking to avoid impulsive action and unwanted outcomes. For example, a response from a target organization may infuriate the advocacy group, stimulating it to rush to the newspapers with its complaint. This may be a good response, it may be playing into the strategy of the target organization, or it may unwittingly drive both sides into an escalated struggle for which the advocacy group may have insufficient resources.

TROUBLESHOOTING

An advocacy action is seldom finished without trouble arising in the conduct of the action. External events occur that could not be anticipated; planned interventions fall short, internal difficulties arise. Some troubles can be attributed to inadequate planning; many cannot be planned for specifically and require skill, knowledge, and experience to resolve as the advocacy action continues.

Some common troubles:

Not enough hands. The advocate doesn't have enough time to do everything he or she has to, or the advocacy group has fallen behind in its assignments. Usually the trouble stems from insufficient delegation of tasks, or from too little participation by others. Or the goals set and the initial plan were too ambitious for the available time.

Second thoughts. Doubts or barriers arise internally after the action is under way. Executive director, board, or staff may raise serious questions about the action. Time may be needed to bring them aboard. Perhaps they were left out originally. The action may have gotten out of control without the advocate realizing it. This type of trouble can be minimized in advance if the agency has a formalized process for selecting advocacy issues and for reviewing plans for action.

Delays. External or internal events may cause delays in the action. Delaying tactics on the part of the target organization can be met by further directed action, and may not affect morale. But other delays may affect the schedule and also the morale of those associated with the advocacy effort. The plan may have to be revised. The advocate or other staff person will probably need to work with individuals, subgroups, or the entire group, in whatever combinations are needed, to maintain morale and to try to use the time constructively.

Interventions fall short or fail. The press release didn't get printed; the public meeting was poorly attended; the telephone campaign failed to elicit much support. Often groundwork was inadequate when interventions fail, but this can happen also for reasons outside one's control. The results should be taken seriously. Failures point to what more needs to be done, calling for revisions in the planning and action. Other failures may be anticipated. For example, in one case a direct appeal was made by letter to the decision maker in the target organization and was denied. This was anticipated, but the move had to be made before further steps could be taken.

Lack of clarity. The advocate may be unclear about his or her role, or the group may become unlcear about goals, with dissension or indecision arising about what to do next.

Power problems. Factional disputes often arise, either on ideological grounds or around leaders vying for power and influence. Supporting groups may compete with each other, or resort to exclusionary tactics. In some situations, a moderate degree of conflict can be channeled into goal-directed behavior instead. In others, the advocacy effort may be seriously disrupted unless the differences can be worked through. The advocate will have to understand the sources of conflict in order to help. In situations such as coalitions, it can happen that one group will be found to be at such variance with the generally accepted goals that the only solution is dropping that group.

Dissatisfied and disruptive individuals. Dissatisfied individuals often drop out, sometimes quietly, sometimes noisily, but usually with some effect on the others. Individualized handling, based on understanding of the person and his or her situation, is called for, preferably before the person drops out, since it is difficult to get someone back and often undesirable to coax him or her. Personal dissatisfaction

may be first evidenced in complaining, express-
ing of doubts in indirect ways, slackening of
effort, unresponsiveness. Disruptive individuals are those who characteristically do not
fit well into groups or work well with others,
or who have abrasive personalities. Sometimes
they can be placed in roles where their drawbacks are minimized and their assets utilized.
Often a group may be unable to tolerate them.
Some disruptive people may be reacting to temporary problems in their own lives, and can be
helped over this period. Others may have to be
eased out, either through personal discussion or
through such devices as reorganizing the structure or redesigning roles. To some extent,
this type of difficulty - dissatisfaction and
disruption - can be avoided if the planning of
goals includes a participation goal; attention
is paid in this goal to the meaning of participation for the individual, and planning of roles
takes this into account. Difficulties should
then emerge early, rather than later, after the
action is under way. Provision for shifting
roles or progression in roles would be part of
the planning.

Individual relationships to the advocacy effort,
group relations, and individual interactions obviously benefit when handled with skill in group dynamics and in working with individuals. The advocate may use other agency staff members as consul-
tants, both in understanding the problem and in
understanding his or her part in it, or may have
other staff members handle certain problems directly.

EVALUATION

Evaluation should be built into the advocacy process from the beginning. Although no systematic methods for evaluation of an advocacy effort are in general use, evaluation is possible in a number of ways.

A first principle is that measuring an advocacy effort by the simple either-or standard of success or failure is misleading. If, in the planning of the effort, goals were established in regard to the problem itself, in regard to participation in the effort, and in regard to the education that occurred, evaluation should take into account the goals that were achieved and those that were missed.

An evaluation of an advocacy effort is important for several reasons. The practitioners will benefit by what they learn. Agency boards and staff will gain a better understanding of advocacy. Funding sources may be better able to fit advocacy into their service definitions and statistics if they have access to evaluations results. Finally, advocacy as a field of activity will be advanced by the knowledge that accrues in evaluation.

Once again, an examination of the methods used in casework will be instructive regarding advocacy. Much of the evaluation of casework is quantitative - the accumulation of statistics: the number of cases, the number of interviews per case,

the types of treatment used, and other service activity data. Qualitative evaluations take the form
of an assessment by the caseworker of the outcomes. A detailed case record provides a running
account of the course of counseling or summarized
recording presents the case by such analytic categories as background, presenting problem, and diagnosis. Another form of evaluation, now being used
by many family agencies, is feedback from consumers, usually elicited through a questionnaire.

Casework evaluations can be adapted to advocacy
in the following ways:

Descriptive evaluations. The log of activities,
often kept by community organizers, is the equi-
valent of the case record. It may also include
copies of fliers, letters, and similar material
that were issued during the advocacy effort.
The log can also contain the advocate's evaluation of the effort.

A topical and analytic description of an advocacy effort might cover such topics as interventions used, constraints encountered, participation, and action steps. This type of evaluation would set forth the goals and conclude with
an evaluation of the results in terms of each.
Baseline data can be included - for example, in
relation to a participation goal, the data might
show an original group of five clients increased
to twenty-five clients and potential clients as
a result of the advocacy effort. Similar "before and after" comparisons can be made in relation to educational and problem goals, without
attempting to accumulate any further data and
analysis.

Feedback from participants. As with casework
clients, feedback can be obtained from advocacy
participants - staff, board, students, volunteers, clients, and consumers, and allied or

supportive groups and organizations. This type of survey can be done simply to obtain reactions of participants without refining the questionnaire further and developing research findings. Such evaluation has the additional value of making participants more aware of the value of their participation to themselves as well as to the issue. A more elaborate survey would involve a "before and after" questionnaire, but would require a sophisticated analysis to be useful.

Statistics. Data on activities can be gathered during the course of advocacy or derived from a log. The data can be categorized in various ways, such as a listing of the people contacted - those within the agency and those outside. A tabulation of the number of contacts with each can be further divided into whether the contacts were with individuals, small groups, or large groups. The reason for each contact could be tabulated. An example of the latter may be found in Promoting Innovation and Change in Organizations and Communities.[1] Data may also be related to each type of goal: problem, participant, and educational.

This analysis would provide accountability for advocacy. It does not, of course, provide measures of quality. Nor could one advocacy effort be compared to another in such quantitative terms - the amount of activity per se does not indicate effectiveness. Such an analysis, however, will provide a quick, graphic presentation of the diversity and complexity of advocacy work.

In summary, evaluation is essential in an advocacy program, to further knowledge and the development of the method, to provide more accountability, and to make the advocacy experience more meaningful for participants.

NOTES

Introduction
1. Robert Sunley, "Family Advocacy: From Case to Cause," Social Casework 51 (June 1970): 347-57.
2. Ellen Manser, ed., Family Advocacy: A Manual for Action (New York: Family Service Association of America, 1973).

Chapter 1
1. Stephen M. Drezner and William B. McCurdy, A Planning Guide for Voluntary Human Service Delivery Agencies (New York: Family Service Association of America, 1973).
2. Salvatore Ambrosino, "Integrating Counseling, Family Life Education, and Family Advocacy," Social Casework 60 (December 1979): 579-85.
3. Jack Rothman, Planning and Organizing for Social Change: Action Principles for Social Science Research (New York: Columbia University Press, 1974); George Brager and Stephen Holloway, Changing Human Service Organizations: Politics and Practice (New York: Free Press, 1978).

Chapter 2
1. Jack Rothman, John L. Erlich, and Joseph G. Teresa, Promoting Innovation and Change in Organizations and Communities: A Planning Manual (New York: John Wiley, 1976).

Chapter 3
1. Robert M. Rice, American Family Policy: Content

and Context (New York: Family Service Association
of America, 1977), p. 79.
2. Robert M. Rice, "Family Policy and Social Work
in the 80s" (Paper delivered at Annual Program
Meeting, Council of Social Work Education, 1980).
3. Drezner and McCurdy, A Planning Guide, chapter 5
and appendices D and E.
4. Standards, National Association of Social Work,
1975, pp. 38-39. See also National Association of
Social Work Ad Hoc Committee on Advocacy, "The
Social Worker as Advocate," pp. 16-22.
5. Family Advocacy Reporter, Nos. 1,2,3 (New York:
Family Service Association of America, 1975, 1976,
1977). Of the 110 reported actions, 52 focused on
local problems only, a few combined actions on both
state and local level. It should be noted that action on a state level may be directed at the executive branch, not only at the legislature. Resort
to state level courts is also possible in order to
bring about statewide change. Conceivably, a change
in state legislation could be sought to apply to
only one city or community, although this does not
seem to have occurred in the reported cases.

Chapter 4
1. This checklist originated with The Health and
Welfare Council of Nassau County, New York.

Chapter 5
1. Everett M. Rogers, Diffusion of Innovations (New
York: Free Press, 1962).
2. Rothman, Planning and Organizing.
3. Ibid., pp. 115-88.
4. Herman Turk, Organizations in Modern Life (San
Francisco: Jossey-Bass, 1977).
5. Peter M. Blau, Bureaucracy in Modern Society
(New York: Random House, 1956).
6. Chris Argyris, Understanding Organization
Behavior (London: Tavistock, 1960); Rensis Likert,
New Patterns of Management (New York: McGraw-Hill,
1961); John B. Miner, Personnel and Industrial

162

Relations: A Managerial Approach (New York: MacMillan, 1969).
7. Drezner and McCurdy, A Planning Guide.
8. Fred Luthans, Organizational Behavior: A Modern Behavioral Approach to Management (New York: McGraw-Hill, 1973).
9. Carel B. Germain, "General Systems Theory and Ego Psychology: An Ecological Perspective," Social Service Review 52 (December 1978): 535-50.
10.Gordon Hearn, ed., The General Systems Approach: Contributions Toward an Holistic Conception of Social Work (New York: Council on Social Work Education, 1969).
11.Carel B. Germain, "An Ecological Perspective in Casework Practice," Social Casework 54 (June 1973): 326.
12.Rothman, Planning and Organizing.
13.Peter M. Blau and W. Richard Scott, Formal Organizations: A Comparative Approach (San Francisco: Chandler, 1962); Gene W. Dalton and Paul R. Lawrence, eds., Organizational Change and Development (Homewood, Ill.: R.D. Irwin, 1970).
14.Rogers, Diffusion of Innovations.
15.Rothman, Planning and Organizing.
16.Ibid., pp. 279-393.
17.Rothman, Erlich, and Teresa, Promoting Innovation and Change, pp. 96-113.

Chapter 6
1. Rogers, Diffusion of Innovations.

Chapter 7
1. Family Advocacy Reporter, nos. 1, 2, and 3.
2. Rothman, Planning and Organizing, pp. 72-75.
3. Institute on Pluralism and Group Identity, American Jewish Committee, A Practical Guide to Coalition Building (New York: 1976).
4. Rothman, Erlich, and Teresa, Promoting Innovation and Change, pp. 22-57.
5. Rothman, Planning and Organizing.
6. Rogers, Diffusion of Innovations.

Chapter 8

1. John Naisbitt, Megatrends: Ten New Directions Transforming Our Lives (New York: Warner Books, 1982), p. 102.

2. Adapted, with permission of the copyright holder, from "Child Welfare Workers and the State Legislative Process," Child Welfare 57 (January 1978): 13-24.

3. United Way of America, Government Relations Manual (Alexandria, Va.: United Way of America, 1982), p. 33.

4. Ibid.

5. Raymond Albert, "Social Work Advocacy in the Regulatory Process," Social Casework 64 (October 1983): 480-81.

6. Sally Y. Orr, "Volunteers as Advocates," Journal of Voluntary Action Research 11 (April-September 1982): 116.

7. John Herbers, "Study Tells How 14 States Responded to Aid Cuts," The New York Times, 8 May 1983.

8. "The OMB Bomb-Throwers," The New York Times, 15 March 1983.

9. United Way of America, Government Relations Manual, p. 19.

10. Orr, "Volunteers as Advocates," 108-17.

Chapter 10

1. Rothman, Erlich, and Teresa, Promoting Innovation and Change, pp. 233-34.

BIBLIOGRAPHY

Values, Family Policy and Study
Lindblom, Charles E. The Policy-Making Process.
    Englewood Cliffs, N.J.: Prentice Hall, 1968.
    One of the basic texts in this field. Deals
    primarily with national and international pol-
    icy, but the analysis of the process applies to
    any level of policy making. Of particular rele-
    vance to advocacy is chapter on "Limits on Pol-
    icy Analysis" with subsections on "Complexity
    and Inadequate Information" and "Difficulties in
    Organizing Goals or Values." Lindblom points
    out four basic ways in which policy is formed:
    by administrative regulation, by legislation, by
    judicial review, and by citizen pressure.
Rice, Robert M. American Family Policy: Content
    and Context. New York: Family Service
    Association of America, 1977.
    Presents an overview of the several aspects of
    family policy, tracing it historically and in
    relation to family functions; describes indica-
    tors of trends in family life. It reviews pro-
    posals made on family policy for this country.
    Provides a good understanding of the values, im-
    plicit and explicit, underlying the social mea-
    sures which are the objects of broad scale
    change efforts and which often impinge nega-
    tively at the local level.
Rossi, Alice S.; Kagan, Jerome; Hareven, Tamara K.;
    eds. The Family. New York: W.W. Norton, 1978.

Collection of studies by a number of leading
writers in the field of family history gives a
perspective on different approaches and aspects
in the field, and offers rationales for the re-
levance of the history of the family to current
social problems and efforts at solving them.

Schorr, Alvin L. "Family Values and Real Life,"
Social Casework 57 (June 1976), 397-404.
Leading writer on family policy discusses broad
national values of critical importance in the
selection or omission of policy measures for
families. Helps advocates and those involved in
selecting advocacy issues for action understand
the value issues involved.

Organizational Theory, Behavior

Bennis, Warren G.; Benne, Kenneth D.; Chin,
Robert. The Planning of Change. New York:
Holt, Rinehart and Winston, 1969 (2nd ed.).
Collection of articles is one of the best over-
views on planning change, although the sociolo-
gical and social psychological approach renders
much of the material too abstract for direct use
in advocacy.

Etzioni, Amitai. A Comparative Analysis of Complex
Organizations. New York: Free Press, 1961.
A classic study in the field of organizational
theory. Analyzes three main types of organizations, classified by the major method of internal compliance with power and leadership structure. For advocates, book provides another tool
for understanding inherent strengths and weaknesses of organizations. Chapter IX is particularly relevant.

Luthans, Fred. Organizational Behavior: A Modern
Behavioral Approach to Management. New York:
McGraw-Hill, 1973.
A comprehensive text on organizational theories,
as well as on the allied fields of motivation,
learning, and personality development, from a
behavioral point of view. Chapter 19 and chap-

ter 20 analyze conflict and change in organizations and the effects on the behavior of the
individuals within the organization. The review
of the decision making process in chapters 9 and
10, and the organizational communication and
control processes in chapters 11 and 12 should
be helpful to the family agency itself as well
as in understanding target organizations.

Polsky, Howard W. "From Claques to Factions:
Subgroups in Organizations." Social Work 23
(March 1978), 94-99.
Interesting analysis of the roles of subgroups -
claques, loyalists, functionaries, cliques,
cabals, factions. Useful for understanding target organizations and possible strategies.

Rogers, Everett M. Diffusion of Innovations. New
York: Free Press, 1962.
Classic study brings together over 500 research
studies from various fields and proposes a number of principles governing the change process.
An excellent summary of those most pertinent to
family advocacy is found in Rothman's book,
Planning and Organizing for Social Change,"
annotated separately.

Zaltman, Gerald; Duncan, Robert; Holbek, Irving.
Innovations and Organizations. New York: John
Wiley, 1973.
Provides a broad view of concepts relating to
innovation within organizations, as expounded by
various writers on the subject. The book is
focussed on the innovations generated within an
organization, but provides understanding about
the difficulties and stages of change and suggests indirectly intervention points for advocacy.

Systems Theory
Germain, Carel B. "General Systems Theory and Ego
Psychology: An Ecological Perspective," Social
Service Review 52 (December 1978), 535-50.
Provides excellent understanding of systems

theory, the ecological theory, and ego psychology, pointing out common bases couched in differing language. For advocates, explanation of the ecological approach is perhaps most helpful and most directly useful in conceptualizing advocacy.

Hearn, Gordon. The General Systems Approach: Contributions Toward an Holistic Concept of Social Work. New York: Council on Social Work Education, 1969.

Early, important collection of articles applying systems approach to social work to develop concepts. Polsky's article, "System as Patient: Client Needs and System Function," attempts to place systems change within the general concepts relating to interchanges between person and environment, as opposed to a static concept in which the person copes with or adjusts to a fixed system. Lathrope's article, "The General Systems Approach in Social Work Practice," includes "social action practice" as one of the fields of social work practice; and provides an understanding of advocacy, or social action practice, as translated into systems concepts and terminology.

Janchill, Mary P. "Systems Concepts in Casework Theory and Practice," Social Casework 50 (February 1969): 74-82.

Good description of key concepts of systems theory, primarily in relation to social casework with individual and family. By implication, article suggests that systems theory emphasizes the importance of external influences upon both functioning and inner psychological states (viewed as individual pathology in psychodynamic theory).

Orcutt, Ben A. "Casework Intervention and the Problems of the Poor," Social Casework 54 (February 1973): 85-95.

Application of systems theory to casework is described, with case example to show intermeshing of individual, family, and institutions in developing plan for the individual and family. Recognizes need for case advocacy as part of change process, but not of cause advocacy as an outgrowth of the individual cases.

Human Service Organizations - Structure, Goals, Innovations

Brager, George and Holloway, Stephen. Changing Human Service Organizations: Politics and Practice. New York: The Free Press, 1978.
A theoretical and practical guide on how to change an organization from within, by service staff below the top management level. While advocates seek to produce change from outside other organizations or systems, they will find this book valuable in understanding change process, the analysis of the factors involved, and the overall strategies and the tactics available.

Drezner, Stephen M. and McCurdy, William B. A Planning Guide for Voluntary Human Service Delivery Agencies. New York: Family Service Association of America, 1979.
The comprehensive work on planning specifically related to family agencies, and the concepts and techniques apply to planning for family advocacy as well as to the total agency. With some adapting, the planning process fits also into the planning of an advocacy action, although lacking many of the necessary specifics. The complexity of the complete planning process outlined points to an ideal rather than practical model, but many adaptions and shortcuts can be taken to tailor applications to specific situations.

Hasenfeld, Yesheshel and English, Richard, eds. Human Service Organizations. Ann Arbor, Michigan: University of Michigan Press, 1974.
Collection of studies provides excellent analyses of "people-changing" organizations, dividing them into two types: treatment and sociali-

zation. Major studies take up the environment, leadership, goals, technology, authority and control, staffing, client relations, interorganizational relations, evaluation of performance, and organizational innovation and change. Provides a needed bridge between organizational theory and the detailed case study of a single organization which might be made in an advocacy action.

Rice, Robert M. "Organizing to Innovate in Social Work." Social Casework 54 (January 1973): 20-26.

Changes are suggested in agency structure, staff functions, and administration to facilitate effective use of newer methods such as advocacy and informal indivdual and group contacts.

Wiehe, Vernon R. "Management by Objectives in a Family Service Agency," Social Casework 54 (March 1973): 42-46.

Written from agency point of view, article describes the process of defining mission of agency, goals and objectives, and process of involving staff.

Advocacy - General

Albert, Raymond. "Social Work Advocacy in the Regulatory Process," Social Casework 64 (October 1983): 473-81.

This article examines a social work role in the regulatory process, indicating key features of administrative authority, discussing the justification for a social work role, and reviewing intervention techniques.

Community Action for Legal Services, Inc. Manual for Welfare Advocates in New York City. New York: 335 Broadway, New York 10013.

A comprehensive manual on welfare, designed for case advocates. Can serve as a model for any agency or group wishing to develop material on case advocacy in regard to welfare laws, regulations, and practices.

Gartner, Alan and Riessman, Frank. Self-Help in the Human Services. San Francisco: Jossey-Bass, 1977.
Many self-help groups have some emphasis on social change, usually around a single focus. Nonetheless, they are potential allies in advocacy. This book gives a broad overview of self-help groups, including a directory.

Hessel, Dieter T. A Social Action Primer. Philadelphia: Westminster Press, 1972.
Last chapter of this book provides a useful analysis of the characteristics and potential strengths of church memberships for participation in advocacy. Author points out that, with some exceptions, churches as organizations will participate only in low-conflictual level activities. Main body of book appeals to people to become involved in change efforts and presents a simplified overview of the advocacy process.

Jacobs, Joseph D. "Social Action as Therapy in a Mental Hospital," Social Work 9 (January 1964): 54-61.
Article focusses on the use of group work in advocating for social change and on the psychological benefits to the individual participant. The latter aspect is regarded narrowly, in relation to the patient population, but article remains one of the very few contributions to this subject in the past 20 years.

O'Connell, Brian. "From Service to Advocacy to Empowerment," Social Casework 59 (April 1978): 195-202.
The author, then director of the Mental Health Association, traces the evolving roles of volunteers, particularly in regard to advocacy. He deplores the emphasis on service at the expense of advocacy, and sees the effective social action agency as being independent, "free to tackle anybody or cooperate with anybody." This stance runs counter to the prevailing trend to accept and use government funding for services,

with the restrictions on advocacy that necessarily follow. Agencies may question the under-
lying premises that independent advocacy is more
important than service and that government funds
are necessarily and always more restrictive than
voluntary funds.

Prigmore, Charles S. "Use of the Coalition in
Legislative Action," Social Work 19 (January
1974): 96-102.

One of the few articles on the use of coalitions, this one advocates broadening the base of
coalitions far beyond the usual social work
framework, enlisting seemingly disparate, even
antagonistic groups. For some agencies, such
coalitions can help to increase the base of
agency support as well.

Rothman, Jack. Planning and Organizing for Social
Change: Action Principles from Social Science
Research. New York: Columbia University Press,
1974.

Foreword by Richard Cloward states, most justly:
"This book is an outstanding demonstration that
social science findings can be codified and
translated in ways which make them of extreme
value to social work and human service practitioners...It is a model for all future efforts
of its kind." The book covers research published in the years 1964-70.

The format presents a generalization, followed
by references, brief annotations of references,
and action guidelines.

Of particular interest are chapters on organization behavior, political and legislative behavior, participation in social change, and innovation. The companion volume, by Rothman,
Erlich, and Teresa, reports on field tests of
several of the generalizations and is of equal
importance.

Rothman, Jack. "Macro Social Work in a Tightening
Economy," Social Work 24 (July 1979): 274-282.

Of particular interest to advocates is section

172

on local initiatives, in which author describes the vast expansion of citizen participation through review boards, planning bodies, and boards of directors, as well as the widespread growth of neighborhood action organizations. While much of this activity has taken place outside of social work, advocates can view these organizations as offering increasingly broad bases for support, alliance, and coalition.

Rothman, Jack; Erlich, John L. and Teresa, Joseph G. Promoting Innovation and Change in Organizations and Communities. A Planning Manual. New York: John Wiley & Sons: 1976.

This book follows upon Rothman's earlier work, Planning and Organizing for Social Change, and merits the status of a classic, certainly for all those seriously interested in advocacy. Selected "action principles" derived from social science research are field tested in real situations, in a variety of social service organizations. Planning, action process, and outcomes are described with liberal quotes from the logs kept by the practitioners. Chapter IV, "Fostering Participation," is of especial interest. The use of logs to produce quantitative data is also of importance in the beginning efforts of advocates to set down on paper what they are doing. By implication, the book indicates a method by which advocates can, in planning, develop principles to be tested in action and so contribute further to the development of knowledge.

Sosin, Michael. "Social Work Advocacy and the Implementation of Legal Mandates." Social Casework 60 (May 1979): 265-273.

Target organizations may evade or subvert laws, usually within legal bounds, and documentation is difficult to obtain. A strategy to improve implementation needs to take into account three factors: the degree of receptivity by the target organization of the law (the extent to which the changes are congruent with goals, values, and structure of the organization); ability (degree to which organization has or can obtain resources necessary to implement law); and vulnerability (degree to which organization can resist sanctions provided in the law for noncompliance). Suggestions and cautions for social work advocates are provided.

Taebel, Delbert A. "Strategies to Make Bureaucrats Responsive," Social Work 17 (July 1972): 38-43.
Thesis of the article is that bureaucrats will become more responsive as client/consumer groups become less dependent upon them. Bureaucrats don't respond significantly to political pressure (including marches, sit-ins, demonstrations, appeals to elected officials), nor does decentralization of bureaucracy produce more responsiveness. Alternatives include: development of competitive services; positive, supportive input to bureaucracies, rather than only negative input; self-help programs, including neighborhood organizations. Article provides a useful conceptualization of the broad rationale for this trend in advocacy.

United Way of America. Government Relations Manual. Alexandria, Va., 1982.
Defines government relations and explains how it functions within the United Way system. Practical advice on action networks, discussion of techniques for lobbying and for building rapport with elected officials.

Weiner, Hyman. "Social Change and Social Group Work Practice," Social Work 9 (July 1964): 106-112.
A plea is made to modify the focus of group work, from an emphasis on personality development to a combined approach of both the psychological and social aspects of human existence. The article goes beyond the goal of social consciousness to that of social action as a primary aim of group work, bringing the social values

down to specificity in setting targets and in advocacy methods to achieve them. For a related article, see entry on Joseph Jacobs.

The National Assembly of National Voluntary Health and Social Welfare Organizations. Working Together - Advocating for Change. New York, 1979.

A manual focussed on problems of youth, but with much general material on advocacy, particularly on involvement, training, and use of volunteers and on specifics of such interventions as speakers' bureaus, telephone campaigns, exhibits, mailings, and public meetings.

Family Advocacy

Ambrosino, Salvatore. "Integrating Counseling, Family Life, Education, and Family Advocacy," Social Casework 60 (December 1979): 579-85.

Article describes the place of family advocacy among family agency services, and advances the concept of the case advocacy service as one of the three main "doors" by which clients enter - others being counseling and family life education. Groups may move into cause advocacy as an outgrowth of their common concerns expressed in group meetings.

Cameron, J. Donald and Talavero, Esther. "An Advocacy Program for Spanish-Speaking People," Social Casework 57 (July 1976): 427-31.

A family agency's experience is described in developing an advocacy program for a Spanish-speaking population, with commentary on some of the constraints and conflicts encountered and engendered in the target community.

Pearl, Gloria and Barr, Douglas H. "Agencies Advocating Together," Social Casework 57 (December 1976): 611-18.

This article, one of the very few on coalitions in social work literature, is useful in discussing the process of forming on-going coalitions and their structures, some of the "lessons

learned," and types of problems tackled. The
use of the workshop as an intervention tool is
also valuable, illustrating its role in increasing awareness of problems, obtaining media coverage, and aiding in development of action.

Sunley, Robert. "Family Advocacy: From Case to
Cause," Social Casework 51 (June 1970): 347-57.
This article, the first on family advocacy, presents the rationale for "case to cause" advocacy, and relates advocacy to the family agency as
one of the major functions on behalf of clients.

Turrini, Patsy. "A Mothers' Center: Research,
Service and Advocacy," Social Work 22 (November
1977): 478-83.
The mothers' center demonstrates the integration
of family advocacy into individual and group
services, with research contributing to both.
Group members advocate for themselves and others
in the group, progress from their own experience
to cause advocacy to benefit others as well.

Evaluation

Brody, Ralph and Krailo, Holly. "An Approach to
Reviewing the Effectiveness of Programs," Social
Work 23 (May 1978): 226-232.
Written from the perspective of the United Way
allocation process, this article suggests factors involved in the measurement of outputs in
relation to objectives. Three main types of
objectives are operating objectives, production
objectives, and impact objectives. This may
provide some guidance in making a presentation
of the results of a family advocacy program.

McCurdy, William B. Program Evaluation: A
Conceptual Tool Kit for Human Service Delivery
Managers. New York: Family Service Association
of America, 1979.
This very short nontechnical guide relates program evaluation to family agencies. Considerable emphasis is laid on the relationship between program planning and program evaluation.

A companion piece to ATE DUE and McCurdy's "A
Planning Guide," annotated in another section of
this bibliography.

Tripodi, Tony; Fellin, Phillip: Epstein, Irwin.
Differential Social Program Evaluation. Itasca,
Ill.: F.E. Peacock, 1978.
The organization of this most helpful text makes
it a guide to the selection and implementation
of various types of evaluations; it relates objectives and questions to the types of evaluations. Three major types of "evaluation strategies" are covered, each with subdivisions: (1)
monitoring, including social accounting, administrative audit, and time and motion studies;
(2) cost-analytic, including general accounting,
cost accounting, cost-benefit analysis, and
cost-effectiveness analysis; and (3) social research, including experiments, surveys, and case
study. Agencies wishing to evaluate their advocacy programs can use this book to help formu-
late the questions they wish answered, the methods by which answers might be obtained, and
the process and cost involved.